METABOLIC CONFUSION DIET FOOD LIST FOR ENDOMORPH SENIORS

The Metabolic Mastery Guide: Beat Your Body's Game with the Ultimate Collection of Foods for Improved Weight Loss

Vincent John Walker

1

DISCLAIMER

This publication is designed to provide competent and reliable information regarding the subject covered. However, the views expressed in this publication are those of the author alone, and should not be taken as expert instruction or professional advice. The reader is responsible for his or her actions. The author hereby disclaims any responsibility or liability whatsoever that is incurred from the use or application of the contents of this publication by the purchaser of the reader. The purchaser or reader is hereby responsible for his or her actions.

Copyright © 2024

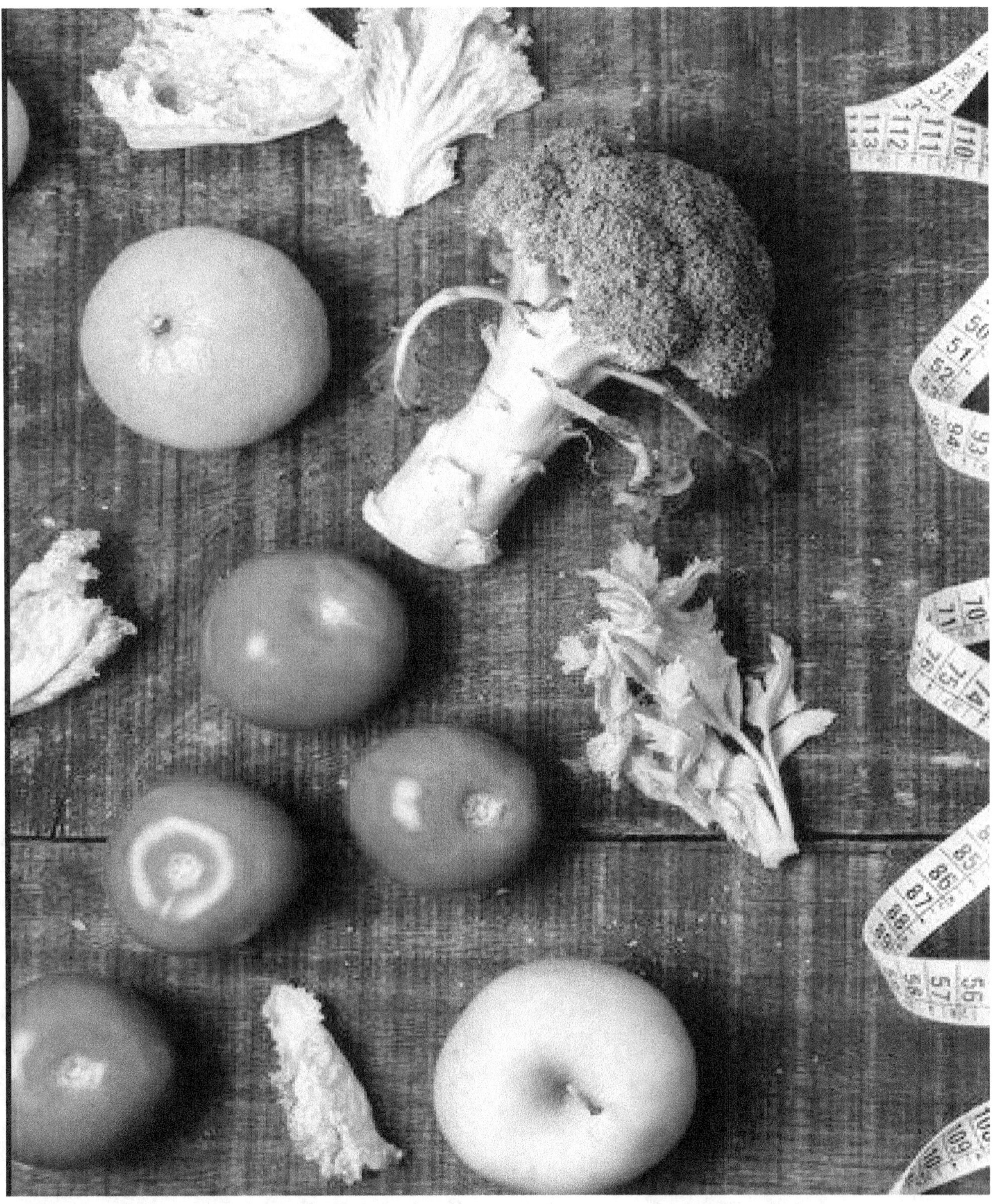

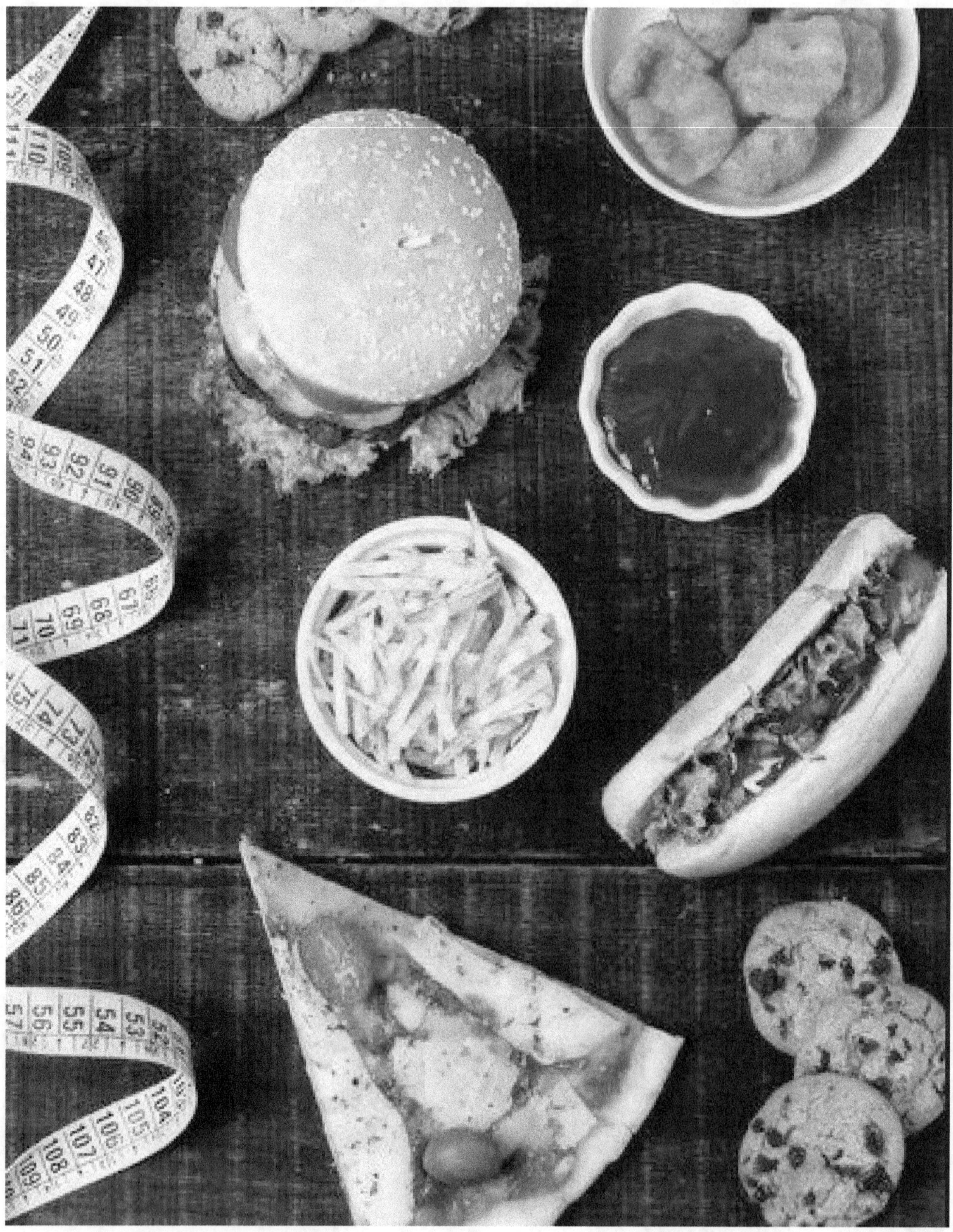

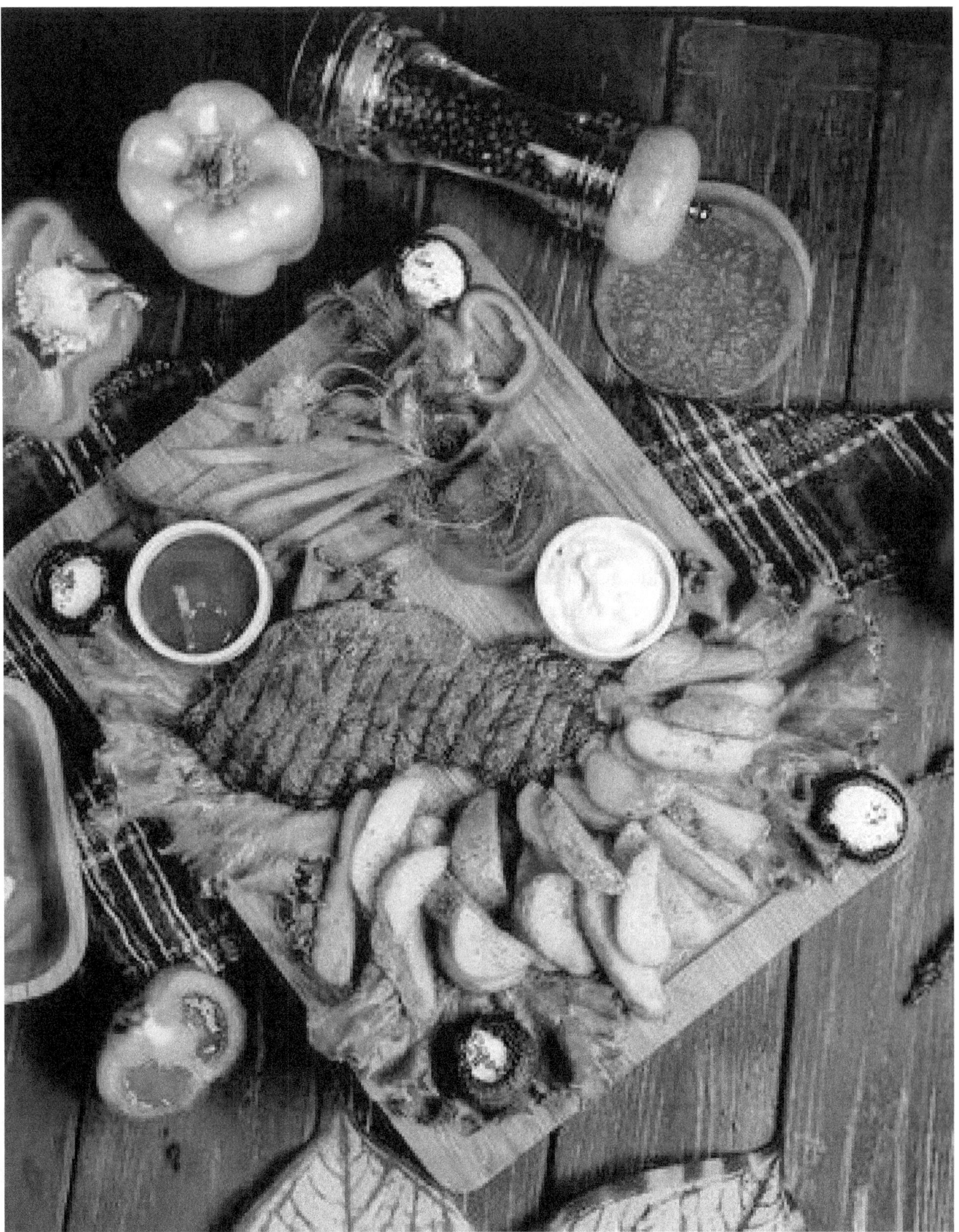

TABLE OF CONTENTS

INTRODUCTION

Welcome to a journey of transformation and empowerment—a journey tailored specifically for you, my dear senior endomorphs. As we embark on this path together, I want you to know that I understand the challenges you face. The frustration of trying various diets, only to see minimal results. The confusion of navigating conflicting information about nutrition and weight loss. The desire to reclaim your health and vitality, but feeling uncertain about where to begin.

But fear not, for within the pages of this book lies a beacon of hope—a roadmap designed to guide you through the intricate landscape of metabolic confusion and empower you to achieve your health and wellness goals.

In a world inundated with fad diets and quick-fix solutions, the Metabolic Confusion Diet offers a refreshing approach—one rooted in science, tailored to your unique physiology, and crafted with the wisdom of years of experience. This is not just another diet; it's a holistic lifestyle shift—a journey towards sustainable health and well-being.

At its core, the Metabolic Confusion Diet recognizes the inherent complexities of the human body, particularly for those of us who identify as endomorphs. We understand that our bodies respond differently to various foods and dietary approaches and that achieving optimal health requires a personalized approach—one that honors our metabolic quirks and challenges.

Throughout this book, we will delve deep into the science behind metabolic confusion, unraveling its mysteries and uncovering its transformative power. We'll explore the intricate dance between metabolism, hormones, and body composition, shedding light on how metabolic confusion can unlock your body's innate potential for weight loss and vitality.

But knowledge alone is not enough; action is required to manifest change. That's why we'll provide you with practical tools and strategies to implement the Metabolic Confusion Diet in your daily life. From designing personalized meal plans to navigating social events and overcoming common challenges, we'll equip you with the skills and confidence you need to succeed.

But perhaps most importantly, this book is a celebration of you—of your resilience, your courage, and your unwavering commitment to your health and well-being. It's a testament to the fact that age is not a barrier to transformation and that with the right guidance and support, you can achieve remarkable results at any stage of life.

So, my fellow endomorph seniors, I invite you to join me on this transformative journey—to embrace the power of metabolic confusion, nourish your body with delicious and nutritious foods, and reclaim your vitality and joy. Together, we'll defy expectations, break free from limitations, and unlock the vibrant, healthy lives we deserve.

Are you ready to embark on this journey? If so, turn the page, and let's begin. Your best self awaits.

How to Use This Book

As you hold this book in your hands, you may be feeling a mix of emotions—excitement, curiosity, perhaps even a touch of apprehension. You've taken the first step on a journey towards better health and well-being, and I commend you for that. However, I understand that embarking on a new dietary regimen can be daunting, especially when faced with the plethora of information and advice available.

That's why I want to reassure you that you're not alone. Throughout the pages of this book, I'll be your guide, your companion, and your cheerleader, offering practical insights and gentle encouragement every step of the way. Together, we'll navigate the complexities of the Metabolic Confusion Diet, demystifying its principles and empowering you to take control of your health.

So, how do you use this book? Let me break it down for you:

Start with an Open Mind: Approach this journey with curiosity and openness. Leave behind any preconceived notions or past experiences with diets. Embrace the opportunity for growth and transformation.

Set Your Intentions: Before diving into the content, take a moment to reflect on your goals and aspirations. What do you hope to achieve with the Metabolic Confusion Diet? Write down your intentions and keep them in mind as you progress through the book.

Engage with the Material: This is not a book to be passively consumed; it's a resource to be engaged with actively. Take notes, highlight key points, and bookmark pages that resonate with you. The more you interact with the material, the deeper your understanding will become.

Take It One Step at a Time: Rome wasn't built in a day, and neither will your health transformation. Pace yourself and focus on making gradual, sustainable changes. Start with small, manageable steps and gradually build momentum over time.

Practice Self-Compassion: Change is hard, and setbacks are inevitable. Be kind to yourself during this process. Celebrate your successes, no matter how small, and learn from your challenges. Remember, progress, not perfection, is the goal.

Stay Connected: You are not alone on this journey. Reach out to friends, family, or online communities for support and accountability. Share your successes, seek advice when needed, and celebrate each other's victories.

Trust the Process: Trust that you have everything you need within you to succeed. Trust in the wisdom of your body and the guidance provided in this book. Trust that with dedication and perseverance, you will achieve your goals.

As you embark on this journey, remember that transformation is not just about the destination—it's about the journey itself. Embrace the challenges, savor the victories, and cherish the moments of growth along the way. You have the power to rewrite your story, and I'm honored to be a part of it.

CHAPTER 1

UNDERSTANDING METABOLISM AND BODY TYPES

Overview of Metabolism

Metabolism is a complex and dynamic process that occurs within the human body to sustain life. It encompasses all the chemical reactions that take place to convert food into energy, which is then utilized by various organs and tissues to perform essential functions such as breathing, circulating blood, and repairing cells. Simply put, metabolism is the rate at which your body burns calories to maintain its basic functions.

Several factors influence metabolism, including age, gender, genetics, body composition, and physical activity level. Basal metabolic rate (BMR) refers to the number of calories your body needs at rest to maintain vital functions. It varies from person to person and is influenced by factors such as muscle mass, age, and hormonal fluctuations.

In addition to BMR, two other components contribute to overall metabolism: the thermic effect of food (TEF) and physical activity level (PAL). TEF refers to the energy expenditure associated with digesting, absorbing, and metabolizing food, while PAL represents the calories burned through physical activity.

Understanding your metabolism is crucial for achieving and maintaining a healthy weight. By adopting lifestyle habits that support a healthy metabolism—such as regular exercise, adequate sleep, and balanced nutrition—you can optimize your body's ability to burn calories efficiently and support overall health and well-being.

The Three Body Types: Ectomorph, Mesomorph, and Endomorph

Humans come in all shapes and sizes, and our body types can be broadly categorized into three main categories: ectomorph, mesomorph, and endomorph. While most individuals exhibit characteristics of more than one body type, one typically predominates, influencing factors such as metabolism, muscle mass, and fat distribution.

Ectomorphs are characterized by a lean and slender build, with a fast metabolism and difficulty gaining weight or muscle mass. They tend to have a high ratio of fast-twitch muscle fibers, which are conducive to endurance activities such as long-distance running or cycling.

Mesomorphs are often described as having a muscular and athletic physique, with a naturally balanced metabolism and the ability to gain muscle and lose fat relatively easily. They typically excel in sports that require strength, power, and agility, such as weightlifting or sprinting.

Endomorphs, on the other hand, have a rounder and softer body shape, with a slower metabolism and a tendency to gain weight, particularly around the abdomen and hips. They may struggle to lose weight despite their best efforts and often find it challenging to maintain a lean physique.

It's essential to recognize that body type is not set in stone and can be influenced by various factors, including genetics, lifestyle habits, and environmental factors. While you may identify more strongly with one body type than the others, it's crucial to focus on embracing and nurturing your unique body, rather than comparing yourself to others.

Identifying Endomorph Characteristics

Endomorphs typically exhibit several distinct physical and metabolic characteristics that set them apart from other body types. These may include:

- A round or pear-shaped body with a tendency to carry excess weight around the abdomen, hips, and thighs.

- Slower metabolism and difficulty losing weight, even with diet and exercise.

- Higher levels of body fat and lower muscle mass compared to ectomorphs and mesomorphs.

- Challenges with insulin sensitivity and blood sugar regulation can contribute to an increased risk of type 2 diabetes and metabolic syndrome.

- Prone to storing fat more easily, particularly in response to excess calorie intake or hormonal fluctuations.

Despite these challenges, endomorphs also possess unique strengths, such as resilience, adaptability, and the ability to excel in activities that require strength and power. By understanding and embracing your endomorphic characteristics, you can develop a personalized approach to nutrition and exercise that supports your health and fitness goals.

Metabolic Challenges for Endomorph Seniors

As we age, our metabolism naturally slows down, leading to a decline in energy expenditure and an increased propensity for weight gain. For endomorph seniors, this metabolic slowdown can pose additional challenges, exacerbating existing difficulties with weight management and body composition.

One significant contributing factor to metabolic challenges in endomorph seniors is a decrease in muscle mass and an increase in body fat percentage. Sarcopenia, or age-related muscle loss, accelerates with advancing age, leading to a decline in metabolic rate and a reduction in overall energy expenditure.

Furthermore, hormonal changes associated with aging, such as declining levels of testosterone and estrogen, can further impact metabolism and body composition. These hormonal shifts can contribute to changes in fat distribution, particularly abdominal obesity, which is associated with an increased risk of metabolic disorders such as type 2 diabetes and cardiovascular disease.

Additionally, age-related changes in lifestyle habits, such as reduced physical activity levels and alterations in dietary patterns, can also influence metabolism and weight management in endomorph seniors. Factors such as decreased mobility, chronic health conditions, and medication use can further complicate the picture, making it challenging to maintain a healthy weight and body composition.

Despite these challenges, there are steps that endomorph seniors can take to support their metabolic health and well-being. Adopting a balanced and nutritious diet, rich in whole foods such as fruits, vegetables, lean proteins, and healthy fats, can provide essential nutrients and support optimal metabolic function. Regular physical activity, including both aerobic exercise and strength training, can help preserve muscle mass, boost metabolism, and improve overall health and vitality.

Moreover, maintaining a healthy weight and body composition is not just about aesthetics—it's about supporting long-term health and well-being. By understanding the unique metabolic challenges faced by endomorph seniors and taking proactive steps to address them, you can optimize your metabolic health and enjoy a vibrant and fulfilling life at any age.

Understanding metabolism and body types is essential for tailoring effective strategies for weight management and overall health. By recognizing and embracing your unique body type, whether you're an endomorph, mesomorph, or ectomorph, you can develop personalized approaches to nutrition, exercise, and lifestyle that support your individual needs and goals. By taking proactive steps to address metabolic challenges and optimize metabolic health, you can enjoy improved energy levels, better physical function, and enhanced overall well-being, regardless of your age or body type.

CHAPTER 2

THE SCIENCE BEHIND METABOLIC CONFUSION

The Concept of Metabolic Confusion

Metabolic confusion is a revolutionary approach to weight loss and metabolic health that challenges conventional wisdom and embraces the complexity of the human body's metabolic processes. At its core, metabolic confusion is based on the principle of disrupting predictable patterns in diet and exercise to prevent metabolic adaptation and promote continuous progress.

The concept of metabolic confusion stems from the recognition that the body is highly adaptive and efficient at maintaining homeostasis, or internal balance, in response to changes in diet and physical activity. When you follow a consistent diet and exercise routine, your body adapts to these stimuli by adjusting its metabolic rate, hormone levels, and energy expenditure to match your intake and activity level.

However, this adaptive response can also hinder weight loss efforts, as the body becomes resistant to further changes and plateaus in progress. Metabolic confusion seeks to disrupt this plateau by introducing periods of variation and unpredictability in diet and exercise, preventing the body from settling into a comfortable equilibrium.

One of the primary mechanisms by which metabolic confusion is achieved is through the manipulation of macronutrient intake and meal timing. By cycling between periods of higher and lower carbohydrate intake, for example, you can keep your body guessing and prevent it from adapting to a specific macronutrient ratio. Similarly, incorporating intermittent fasting or alternate-day fasting can introduce periods of caloric restriction, further enhancing metabolic flexibility and promoting fat loss.

In addition to dietary strategies, varying your exercise routine can also play a crucial role in metabolic confusion. Incorporating a mix of cardiovascular exercise, strength training, and high-intensity interval training (HIIT) can challenge different energy systems and muscle groups, preventing adaptation and promoting continuous progress.

Overall, the concept of metabolic confusion represents a paradigm shift in our understanding of weight loss and metabolic health. Rather than adhering to rigid dietary rules or exercise regimens, metabolic confusion encourages flexibility, variation, and experimentation, allowing individuals to find the approach that works best for their unique physiology and preferences.

How Metabolic Confusion Aids Weight Loss

Metabolic confusion offers a unique approach to weight loss that leverages the body's adaptive nature to maximize fat burning and optimize metabolic health. By introducing periods of variation and unpredictability in diet and exercise, metabolic confusion prevents the body from settling into a comfortable equilibrium, forcing it to continuously adapt and expend energy.

One of the key ways in which metabolic confusion aids weight loss is by preventing metabolic adaptation. When you follow a consistent diet and exercise routine, your body becomes efficient at utilizing energy and conserving calories, making it harder to lose weight over time. Metabolic confusion disrupts this adaptation by introducing changes in diet composition, meal timing, and exercise intensity, keeping the body guessing and preventing it from settling into a plateau.

Moreover, metabolic confusion promotes metabolic flexibility, the body's ability to switch between different fuel sources (such as glucose and fatty acids) in response to changing metabolic demands. By cycling between periods of higher and lower carbohydrate intake, for example, you can train your body to become more efficient at burning fat for fuel, leading to greater fat loss and improved metabolic health.

Furthermore, metabolic confusion enhances calorie expenditure by incorporating periods of caloric restriction or intermittent fasting. By alternating between periods of eating and fasting, you can create a calorie deficit that promotes fat loss while preserving lean muscle mass. Additionally, incorporating varied and challenging exercise routines can further increase energy expenditure and promote fat burning, leading to accelerated weight loss results.

Overall, metabolic confusion offers a flexible and sustainable approach to weight loss that promotes metabolic flexibility, prevents adaptation, and enhances calorie expenditure. By incorporating principles of metabolic confusion into your lifestyle, you can achieve lasting results and optimize your metabolic health for long-term success.

Metabolic Confusion vs. Traditional Diets

Metabolic confusion represents a departure from traditional dieting approaches that rely on rigid rules, calorie counting, and restrictive eating patterns. Unlike traditional diets, which often focus on reducing calories or eliminating specific food groups, metabolic confusion embraces flexibility, variation, and experimentation, allowing individuals to find the approach that works best for their unique physiology and preferences.

One of the key differences between metabolic confusion and traditional diets is the emphasis on macronutrient cycling and meal timing. While traditional diets may prescribe a fixed macronutrient ratio or meal schedule, metabolic confusion encourages variation and unpredictability, cycling between periods of higher and lower carbohydrate intake, for example, or incorporating intermittent fasting protocols. By keeping the body guessing and preventing adaptation, metabolic confusion promotes greater fat loss and metabolic flexibility compared to traditional dieting approaches.

Moreover, metabolic confusion offers a more sustainable and enjoyable approach to weight loss, as it allows for greater flexibility and freedom in food choices. Rather than restricting certain foods or food groups, metabolic confusion encourages a balanced and varied diet that includes a wide range of nutrient-dense foods. This not only supports metabolic health but also promotes long-term adherence and compliance, reducing the likelihood of rebound weight gain or yo-yo dieting.

Additionally, metabolic confusion emphasizes the importance of regular physical activity and exercise in promoting weight loss and metabolic health. While traditional diets may focus solely on calorie restriction, metabolic confusion recognizes the synergistic relationship between diet and exercise, incorporating varied and challenging workout routines to enhance calorie expenditure and promote fat burning.

Overall, metabolic confusion offers a refreshing and effective alternative to traditional dieting approaches, promoting metabolic flexibility, preventing adaptation, and enhancing long-term adherence and compliance. By embracing flexibility, variation, and experimentation, individuals can achieve lasting results and optimize their metabolic health for improved overall well-being.

CHAPTER 3

HEALTH CONSIDERATIONS FOR ENDOMORPH SENIORS

Common Health Concerns in Senior Years

As we age, our bodies undergo a series of changes that can increase the risk of various health concerns. Endomorph seniors, in particular, may face unique challenges related to their body composition and metabolism. Some of the most common health concerns in senior years include:

- **Cardiovascular Disease:** Seniors are at increased risk of developing cardiovascular disease, including heart disease, stroke, and hypertension. Endomorph seniors, who may have higher levels of body fat and lower muscle mass, may be particularly susceptible to these conditions.

- **Type 2 Diabetes:** Age-related changes in metabolism and insulin sensitivity can increase the risk of type 2 diabetes in seniors. Endomorph seniors, who may already have challenges with insulin resistance and blood sugar regulation, may be at even greater risk.

- **Osteoporosis:** Decreased bone density and increased risk of fractures are common concerns for seniors, particularly postmenopausal women. Endomorph seniors may be at higher risk of osteoporosis due to factors such as reduced physical activity and hormonal changes.

- **Arthritis:** Arthritis, including osteoarthritis and rheumatoid arthritis, is prevalent among seniors and can cause pain, stiffness, and reduced mobility. Endomorph seniors may experience additional challenges due to excess weight placing strain on joints.

- **Cognitive Decline:** Age-related cognitive decline, including conditions such as Alzheimer's disease and dementia, is a significant concern for seniors. Maintaining a healthy lifestyle, including regular physical activity and a balanced diet, is crucial for preserving cognitive function.

Nutritional Needs of Seniors

Nutrition plays a critical role in supporting overall health and well-being, especially as we age. Endomorph seniors, in particular, may have unique nutritional needs and challenges related to their body composition and metabolism. Some key considerations for meeting the nutritional needs of endomorph seniors include:

- **Adequate Protein Intake:** Protein is essential for maintaining muscle mass, bone health, and overall vitality, especially in seniors. Endomorph seniors may benefit from slightly higher protein intake to support muscle maintenance and repair.

- **Healthy Fats:** While it's essential to limit saturated and trans fats, healthy fats such as omega-3 fatty acids are crucial for heart health, brain function, and inflammation control. Incorporating sources of healthy fats such as fatty fish, nuts, seeds, and avocado can support overall health and well-being.

- **Fiber-Rich Foods:** Adequate fiber intake is essential for digestive health, weight management, and blood sugar control. Endomorph seniors may benefit from increasing their intake of fiber-rich foods such as fruits, vegetables, whole grains, and legumes to support satiety and promote regularity.

- **Micronutrient-Rich Foods:** Seniors may have increased nutrient needs due to factors such as reduced absorption and utilization of nutrients. Endomorph seniors should focus on consuming a variety of nutrient-dense foods, including fruits, vegetables, whole grains, lean proteins, and dairy or dairy alternatives, to ensure they meet their daily nutrient requirements.

- **Hydration:** Dehydration is a common concern for seniors and can contribute to a range of health issues, including urinary tract infections, kidney stones, and cognitive decline. Endomorph seniors should prioritize staying hydrated by drinking plenty of fluids throughout the day, especially water and other low-calorie beverages.

In addition to meeting nutritional needs, endomorph seniors should also consider factors such as portion control, meal timing, and food quality when planning their diets.

Adjusting for Reduced Mobility and Activity Levels

Maintaining mobility and physical activity is crucial for overall health and well-being, especially as we age. However, endomorph seniors may face challenges related to reduced mobility and activity levels, which can impact their ability to stay active and independent. Some strategies for adjusting to reduced mobility and activity levels include:

- **Focus on Low-Impact Activities:** Endomorph seniors with mobility issues may benefit from low-impact activities such as walking, swimming, cycling, or tai chi, which can help improve cardiovascular health, muscle strength, and flexibility without placing excessive strain on joints.

- **Incorporate Strength Training:** Strength training exercises are essential for preserving muscle mass, bone density, and functional independence in seniors. Endomorph seniors can benefit from incorporating resistance exercises such as bodyweight exercises, resistance bands, or light weights into their routine to maintain muscle strength and mobility.

- **Stay Active Throughout the Day:** Encouraging movement and activity throughout the day can help offset the negative effects of prolonged sitting and sedentary behavior. Endomorph seniors should aim to break up long periods of sitting with short bursts of activity, such as stretching, walking, or gardening, to improve circulation and maintain mobility.

- **Seek Professional Guidance:** Seniors with mobility issues or chronic health conditions should consult with a healthcare professional or physical therapist before starting a new exercise program. They can provide personalized recommendations and guidance to ensure safe and effective exercise participation.

- **Make Environmental Modifications:** Modifying the home environment to support mobility and safety can help endomorph seniors maintain independence and reduce the risk of falls and injuries. Simple modifications such as installing handrails, removing trip hazards, and using assistive devices can make a significant difference in seniors' ability to move around their homes safely.

Medications and Nutrient Absorption

Many seniors take medications to manage chronic health conditions, alleviate symptoms, or improve their quality of life. However, certain medications can affect nutrient absorption, metabolism, and overall nutritional status, which may have implications for endomorph seniors' health and well-being. Some common medications and their potential effects on nutrient absorption include:

- **Proton Pump Inhibitors (PPIs):** PPIs are commonly used to treat gastroesophageal reflux disease (GERD) and other digestive disorders by reducing stomach acid production. However, long-term use of PPIs has been associated with reduced absorption of nutrients such as vitamin B12, calcium, magnesium, and iron, which can lead to deficiencies and related health issues.

- **Statins:** Statins are medications used to lower cholesterol levels and reduce the risk of heart disease and stroke. While statins are generally safe and effective, they can interfere with the production of coenzyme Q10 (CoQ10), a compound involved in energy production and antioxidant defense. CoQ10 supplementation may be beneficial for endomorph seniors taking statins to mitigate potential side effects.

- **Diuretics:** Diuretics, also known as water pills, are commonly used to treat high blood pressure, heart failure, and edema by increasing urine production and reducing fluid retention. However, diuretics can deplete electrolytes such as potassium, magnesium, and calcium, which are essential for muscle function, heart health, and bone density. Endomorph seniors taking diuretics may need to monitor their electrolyte levels and supplement as necessary.

- **Metformin:** Metformin is a medication commonly used to treat type 2 diabetes by lowering blood sugar levels and improving insulin sensitivity. However, long-term use of metformin has been associated with reduced vitamin B12 absorption, which can lead to deficiency and related neurological symptoms. Endomorph seniors taking metformin may benefit from regular monitoring of vitamin B12 levels and supplementation if necessary.

Endomorph seniors need to be aware of the potential effects of medications on nutrient absorption and overall nutritional status.

By prioritizing a balanced and varied diet, staying active and mobile, and monitoring medication use, endomorph seniors can maintain optimal health and vitality in their senior years.

CHAPTER 4

DESIGNING YOUR METABOLIC CONFUSION DIET

Principles of the Metabolic Confusion Diet

The Metabolic Confusion Diet is a dynamic and flexible approach to nutrition that harnesses the power of metabolic variability to promote fat loss, enhance metabolic health, and support overall well-being. Unlike traditional diets that rely on rigid rules and calorie counting, the Metabolic Confusion Diet emphasizes variation, flexibility, and intuition, allowing individuals to tailor their dietary approach to their unique needs and preferences.

At its core, the Metabolic Confusion Diet is guided by several key principles:

- Variation: The cornerstone of the Metabolic Confusion Diet is variation in both diet and exercise. By introducing periods of variation and unpredictability, the body is prevented from adapting to a specific dietary or exercise regimen, promoting continuous progress and preventing plateaus.

- Flexibility: The Metabolic Confusion Diet prioritizes flexibility and adaptability, allowing individuals to adjust their dietary approach based on factors such as hunger, energy levels, and lifestyle preferences. Rather than adhering to strict meal plans or food rules, individuals are encouraged to listen to their bodies and make choices that support their overall health and well-being.

- Balance: A balanced approach to nutrition is essential for long-term success in the Metabolic Confusion Diet. Rather than demonizing specific foods or food groups, the diet emphasizes the importance of including a variety of nutrient-dense foods in moderation, including fruits, vegetables, lean proteins, healthy fats, and whole grains.

- Mindful Eating: Mindful eating is a key component of the Metabolic Confusion Diet, encouraging individuals to slow down, savor their food, and pay attention to hunger and fullness cues. By practicing mindful eating, individuals can develop a healthier relationship with food, improve digestion, and prevent overeating.

Calculating Your Caloric Needs

Understanding your caloric needs is essential for designing an effective Metabolic Confusion Diet that supports your weight loss and metabolic goals. While traditional approaches to calorie counting can be tedious and unsustainable, there are simpler methods for estimating your caloric needs that can provide a useful starting point.

One common method for calculating caloric needs is the Harris-Benedict equation, which takes into account your age, gender, weight, height, and activity level to estimate your basal metabolic rate (BMR)—the number of calories your body needs at rest to maintain vital functions. From there, you can apply an activity factor to estimate your total daily energy expenditure (TDEE), which represents the number of calories you need to maintain your current weight.

Once you have calculated your TDEE, you can adjust your calorie intake based on your weight loss goals. To lose weight, you will need to create a calorie deficit by consuming fewer calories than your TDEE. A moderate calorie deficit of 500 to 750 calories per day is generally recommended for safe and sustainable weight loss, resulting in a loss of approximately 1 to 1.5 pounds per week.

It's important to note that individual calorie needs can vary based on factors such as metabolism, muscle mass, and hormonal fluctuations. Additionally, the accuracy of calorie calculations may be limited by factors such as variations in metabolic rate and activity levels.

While calorie counting can be a useful tool for weight management, it's essential to approach it with flexibility and mindfulness. Rather than obsessing over every calorie, focus on adopting a balanced and varied diet that supports your overall health and well-being. By listening to your body and making choices that align with your hunger and fullness cues, you can achieve lasting success on your Metabolic Confusion Diet journey.

Macronutrient Ratios for Endomorphs

Macronutrient ratios play a crucial role in the Metabolic Confusion Diet, influencing factors such as energy levels, satiety, and metabolic rate. While there is no one-size-fits-all approach to macronutrient ratios, endomorphs may benefit from specific recommendations tailored to their unique physiology and metabolic needs.

One common macronutrient ratio for endomorphs on the Metabolic Confusion Diet is the "40/30/30" ratio, which consists of 40% carbohydrates, 30% protein, and 30% fat. This ratio provides a balanced approach to nutrition, supporting energy levels, muscle maintenance, and overall metabolic health.

Carbohydrates are the body's primary source of energy and play a crucial role in fueling physical activity and supporting brain function. Endomorphs may benefit from focusing on complex carbohydrates such as whole grains, fruits, vegetables, and legumes, which provide sustained energy and promote satiety.

Protein is essential for muscle maintenance, repair, and growth, especially for endomorphs who may have higher levels of body fat and lower muscle mass. Including lean protein sources such as poultry, fish, eggs, dairy, tofu, and legumes in each meal can help support muscle maintenance, promote satiety, and enhance metabolic rate.

Fat is a crucial nutrient for hormone production, cell membrane function, and nutrient absorption. Endomorphs may benefit from focusing on healthy fats such as monounsaturated and polyunsaturated fats found in nuts, seeds, avocados, olive oil, and fatty fish. These fats provide essential nutrients and promote feelings of fullness, which can help prevent overeating and support weight loss.

While the "40/30/30" ratio is a common starting point for endomorphs on the Metabolic Confusion Diet, it's essential to listen to your body and adjust your macronutrient intake based on factors such as hunger, energy levels, and metabolic goals. Experimenting with different ratios and observing how your body responds can help you find the approach that works best for you.

Creating a Flexible Meal Plan

Creating a flexible meal plan is essential for success on the Metabolic Confusion Diet, allowing you to balance your nutritional needs, preferences, and lifestyle. Rather than following a rigid meal plan or set of rules, aim to develop a framework that supports your overall health and well-being while allowing for variation and spontaneity.

Start by identifying your nutritional needs and preferences, including your calorie and macronutrient goals, dietary restrictions, and food preferences. From there, brainstorm a list of nutritious and delicious foods that you enjoy and that align with your goals, such as lean proteins, whole grains, fruits, vegetables, and healthy fats.

Once you have a list of foods to choose from, you can start planning your meals and snacks for the week ahead. Aim to include a balance of carbohydrates, proteins, and fats in each meal, along with plenty of fruits and vegetables for added nutrients and fiber.

To add variety and prevent boredom, experiment with different recipes, cuisines, and cooking methods. Batch cooking and meal prep can also be useful strategies for saving time and ensuring that nutritious meals are readily available throughout the week.

Flexibility is key when it comes to meal planning on the Metabolic Confusion Diet. Rather than rigidly adhering to a set meal plan, be open to changes and adjustments based on factors such as hunger, energy levels, and social occasions. Listen to your body, honor your hunger and fullness cues, and make choices that support your overall health and well-being.

CHAPTER 5

THE METABOLIC CONFUSION FOOD LIST

Overview of Food Categories

Understanding the different food categories is crucial when crafting a diet that aligns with the principles of the Metabolic Confusion plan. By diversifying your food intake across various categories, you ensure that your nutritional requirements are met while promoting metabolic health and aiding in weight loss.

Let's break down the key food categories and the benefits they offer:

1. **Protein:** Proteins are essential macronutrients vital for maintaining, repairing, and growing muscles. Adequate protein intake supports feelings of fullness, helps regulate blood sugar levels, and contributes to the development of lean body mass. Great sources of protein include lean meats like chicken, turkey, and fish, as well as plant-based options such as tofu, tempeh, legumes, and nuts.

2. **Carbohydrates:** Carbohydrates serve as the body's primary energy source, fueling physical activities and supporting brain function. However, not all carbs are equal. Complex carbohydrates, found in whole grains, fruits, vegetables, and legumes, provide sustained energy and promote satiety, while simple carbohydrates like candy, soda, and baked goods can lead to blood sugar spikes and energy crashes.

3. **Fats:** Healthy fats play critical roles in hormone production, cell function, and nutrient absorption. Incorporating sources of healthy fats such as avocados, nuts, seeds, olive oil, and fatty fish into your diet supports heart health, cognitive function, and inflammation regulation. Opt for unsaturated fats over saturated and trans fats whenever possible to optimize overall well-being.

4. **Vegetables:** Vegetables are packed with essential vitamins, minerals, antioxidants, and fiber, making them indispensable for overall health. Aim to include a variety of colorful vegetables

in your meals, including leafy greens, cruciferous veggies, root vegetables, and nightshades. A diverse array of vegetables ensures you receive a broad spectrum of nutrients to bolster metabolic health and immune function.

5. **Fruits:** Like vegetables, fruits offer an abundance of vitamins, minerals, antioxidants, and fiber, making them valuable additions to your diet. However, fruits also contain natural sugars, so moderation is key, especially for weight management and blood sugar control. Opt for whole fruits over juices or dried varieties to maximize fiber intake and minimize sugar content.

6. **Dairy and Alternatives:** Dairy products like milk, yogurt, and cheese provide calcium, protein, and other essential nutrients. For those who are lactose intolerant or follow a plant-based diet, numerous dairy alternatives are available, including almond milk, soy milk, coconut yogurt, and cashew cheese. Choose unsweetened and fortified options to reap the nutritional benefits.

7. **Grains and Grain Alternatives:** Whole grains such as brown rice, quinoa, oats, and barley offer fiber, vitamins, minerals, and antioxidants, supporting metabolic health and weight loss. If you're gluten intolerant or prefer a low-carb approach, consider alternatives like cauliflower rice, zucchini noodles, or almond flour.

8. Beverages: Hydration is vital for overall well-being, so prioritize fluids throughout the day. Water is the best choice, but herbal teas, sparkling water, and coconut water also offer hydration. Limit consumption of sugary drinks like soda, fruit juice, and sports beverages, as they can contribute to weight gain and metabolic issues.

Protein: Building Blocks for Muscle

Food Name	Portion Size	Calories (kcal)	Carbohydrates (g)	Protein (g)	Fat (g)	Fiber (g)	Vitamins & Minerals

Chicken Breast	3 oz	165	0	31	3.6	0	Vitamin B6, Phosphorus, Selenium
Turkey Breast	3 oz	125	0	26	1	0	Vitamin B6, Niacin, Phosphorus, Selenium
Salmon	3 oz	177	0	23	9.7	0	Vitamin D, Vitamin B12, Omega-3 Fatty Acids
Tuna	3 oz	99	0	22	0.9	0	Vitamin D, Vitamin B12, Selenium
Tilapia	3 oz	111	0	23	2.3	0	Vitamin B12, Phosphorus, Selenium
Cod	3 oz	70	0	15	0.7	0	Vitamin B12, Phosphorus, Selenium
Shrimp	3 oz	84	0	18	0.9	0	Vitamin B12, Iron, Magnesium
Beef (Lean Sirloin)	3 oz	162	0	26	5.9	0	Vitamin B12, Iron, Zinc

Pork Tenderloin	3 oz	122	0	22	3.2	0	Vitamin B6, Thiamine, Selenium
Ground Beef (90% lean)	3 oz	184	0	22	10	0	Vitamin B12, Iron, Zinc
Eggs	1 large	72	0.4	6	4.8	0	Vitamin D, Vitamin B12, Selenium, Choline
Greek Yogurt (Plain)	1 cup	154	6	17	8.6	0	Calcium, Vitamin B12, Phosphorus, Potassium
Cottage Cheese	1/2 cup	104	3.5	14	4	0	Calcium, Vitamin B12, Phosphorus
Tofu	3 oz	52	2	6	2.7	0	Calcium, Iron, Magnesium
Tempeh	3 oz	162	9	15	9.4	0	Calcium, Iron, Magnesium
Lentils	1/2 cup	115	20	9	0.4	8	Folate, Iron, Potassium
Chickpeas	1/2 cup	134	23	7	2.1	6	Folate, Iron, Magnesium

Black Beans	1/2 cup	114	20	7	0.5	8	Folate, Iron, Magnesium
Kidney Beans	1/2 cup	112	20	7.7	0.3	6.4	Folate, Iron, Magnesium
Quinoa	1/2 cup	111	19	4	1.8	2.6	Iron, Magnesium, Phosphorus
Chia Seeds	1 oz	138	12	4.7	8.7	9.8	Calcium, Iron, Magnesium
Hemp Seeds	1 oz	162	3	9.2	12.6	1.2	Calcium, Iron, Magnesium
Pumpkin Seeds	1 oz	151	5	7	13	1.7	Magnesium, Phosphorus, Manganese
Almonds	1 oz	164	6	6	14	3.5	Vitamin E, Magnesium, Riboflavin
Peanut Butter	2 tbsp	188	6	8	16	2	Vitamin E, Niacin, Magnesium, Phosphorus
Chickpea Pasta	2 oz	180	32	10	2	8	Iron, Magnesium, Phosphorus

Turkey Bacon	2 slices	60	0	6	3	0	Niacin, Vitamin B6, Selenium
Edamame	1/2 cup	120	9	11	5	4	Folate, Vitamin K, Iron
Seitan	3 oz	120	4	24	0.5	0	Iron, Calcium, Phosphorus
Cottage Cheese	1/2 cup	104	3.5	14	4	0	Calcium, Vitamin B12, Phosphorus
Greek Yogurt (Plain)	1 cup	154	6	17	8.6	0	Calcium, Vitamin B12, Phosphorus, Potassium
Lentils	1/2 cup	115	20	9	0.4	8	Folate, Iron, Potassium
Chickpeas	1/2 cup	134	23	7	2.1	6	Folate, Iron, Magnesium
Black Beans	1/2 cup	114	20	7	0.5	8	Folate, Iron, Magnesium
Kidney Beans	1/2 cup	112	20	7.7	0.3	6.4	Folate, Iron, Magnesium
Quinoa	1/2 cup	111	19	4	1.8	2.6	Iron, Magnesium, Phosphorus

Chia Seeds	1 oz	138	12	4.7	8.7	9.8	Calcium, Iron, Magnesium
Hemp Seeds	1 oz	162	3	9.2	12.6	1.2	Calcium, Iron, Magnesium
Pumpkin Seeds	1 oz	151	5	7	13	1.7	Magnesium, Phosphorus, Manganese
Almonds	1 oz	164	6	6	14	3.5	Vitamin E, Magnesium, Riboflavin
Peanut Butter	2 tbsp	188	6	8	16	2	Vitamin E, Niacin, Magnesium, Phosphorus
Chickpea Pasta	2 oz	180	32	10	2	8	Iron, Magnesium, Phosphorus
Turkey Bacon	2 slices	60	0	6	3	0	Niacin, Vitamin B6, Selenium
Edamame	1/2 cup	120	9	11	5	4	Folate, Vitamin K, Iron
Seitan	3 oz	120	4	24	0.5	0	Iron, Calcium, Phosphorus

Carbohydrates: Energy Sources

Food Name	Portion Size	Calories (kcal)	Carbohydrates (g)	Protein (g)	Fat (g)	Fiber (g)	Vitamins & Minerals
Brown Rice	1/2 cup	108	22	2	0.5	1.8	Magnesium, Manganese, Selenium, B Vitamins
Quinoa	1/2 cup	111	19	4	1.8	2.6	Magnesium, Phosphorus, Folate, Iron
Oats	1/2 cup	150	27	5	3	4	Manganese, Phosphorus, Magnesium, Vitamin B1
Sweet Potato	1 medium	112	26	2	0.1	3.9	Vitamin A, Vitamin C, Manganese, Fiber
Quinoa	1/2 cup	111	19	4	1.8	2.6	Magnesium, Phosphorus, Folate, Iron
Barley	1/2 cup	97	21	3	0.4	3	Manganese, Selenium, Copper, Vitamin B1

Whole Wheat Bread	1 slice	69	12	3	1	1.9	Selenium, Manganese, Fiber, Phosphorus
Spaghetti (Whole Wheat)	1/2 cup	87	19	4	0.5	3	Manganese, Selenium, Phosphorus, Fiber
Buckwheat	1/2 cup	154	33	6	1	4.5	Manganese, Magnesium, Copper, Fiber
Millet	1/2 cup	207	41	6	1.7	2.3	Magnesium, Phosphorus, Copper, Vitamin B1
Amaranth	1/2 cup	125	23	4	1.9	2.6	Calcium, Iron, Phosphorus, Vitamin B6
Bulgur	1/2 cup	76	17	3	0.2	4	Manganese, Magnesium, Fiber, Vitamin B6
Whole Grain Pasta	1/2 cup	99	20	3	0.5	2	Manganese, Selenium, Phosphorus, Fiber

Wild Rice	1/2 cup	101	21	3	0.3	1.3	Magnesium, Phosphorus, Manganese, Vitamin B6
Rye	1/2 cup	208	43	9	1.6	4.1	Manganese, Magnesium, Phosphorus, Fiber
Whole Grain Crackers	1 serving	120	20	2	4	3	Iron, Magnesium, Selenium, Fiber
Popcorn	1 cup	31	6	1	0.4	1.2	Manganese, Magnesium, Phosphorus, Fiber
Buckwheat Flour	1/2 cup	326	71	12	2.3	8	Iron, Magnesium, Phosphorus, Niacin
Farro	1/2 cup	340	73	12	2	7	Magnesium, Zinc, Iron, Vitamin B3
Corn	1/2 cup	60	15	2	0.5	1.5	Vitamin C, Magnesium, Phosphorus, Fiber

Whole Grain Cereal	1 cup	124	26	4	1	5	Iron, Zinc, Magnesium, Vitamin B12
Bulgar Wheat	1/2 cup	150	34	6	1	8	Magnesium, Phosphorus, Niacin, Folate
Whole Grain Tortilla	1 medium	128	22	4	2.5	3	Calcium, Iron, Magnesium, Phosphorus
Buckwheat Pasta	1/2 cup	210	41	8	1.7	4.5	Manganese, Magnesium, Copper, Fiber
Whole Wheat Couscous	1/2 cup	111	24	4	0.4	2	Magnesium, Phosphorus, Folate, Vitamin B1
Popcorn	1 cup	31	6	1	0.4	1.2	Manganese, Magnesium, Phosphorus, Fiber
Buckwheat Flour	1/2 cup	326	71	12	2.3	8	Iron, Magnesium, Phosphorus, Niacin
Farro	1/2 cup	340	73	12	2	7	Magnesium, Zinc, Iron, Vitamin B3

Corn	1/2 cup	60	15	2	0.5	1.5	Vitamin C, Magnesium, Phosphorus, Fiber
Whole Grain Cereal	1 cup	124	26	4	1	5	Iron, Zinc, Magnesium, Vitamin B12
Bulgar Wheat	1/2 cup	150	34	6	1	8	Magnesium, Phosphorus, Niacin, Folate
Whole Grain Tortilla	1 medium	128	22	4	2.5	3	Calcium, Iron, Magnesium, Phosphorus
Buckwheat Pasta	1/2 cup	210	41	8	1.7	4.5	Manganese, Magnesium, Copper, Fiber
Whole Wheat Couscous	1/2 cup	111	24	4	0.4	2	Magnesium, Phosphorus, Folate, Vitamin B1

Fats: Essential Nutrients

Food Name	Portion Size	Calories (kcal)	Carbohydrates (g)	Protein (g)	Fat (g)	Fiber (g)	Vitamins & Minerals
Avocado	1/2 medium	161	8.6	2	15	6.7	Vitamin K, Folate, Vitamin C, Potassium

Olive Oil	1 tbsp	119	0	0	13.5	0	Vitamin E, Vitamin K, Antioxidants
Coconut Oil	1 tbsp	121	0	0	13.5	0	Lauric Acid, Medium-Chain Triglycerides, Antioxidants
Almonds	1 oz	164	6	6	14	3.5	Vitamin E, Magnesium, Riboflavin
Walnuts	1 oz	185	4	4	18.5	2	Omega-3 Fatty Acids, Vitamin E, Antioxidants
Chia Seeds	1 oz	138	12	4.7	8.7	9.8	Calcium, Iron, Magnesium
Flaxseeds	1 tbsp	37	1.6	1.3	3	1.9	Omega-3 Fatty Acids, Fiber, Vitamin B1
Sunflower Seeds	1 oz	164	6	5	14.2	2.4	Vitamin E, Copper, Magnesium
Pumpkin Seeds	1 oz	151	5	7	13	1.7	Magnesium, Phosphorus, Manganese
Peanut Butter	2 tbsp	188	6	8	16	2	Vitamin E, Niacin,

						Magnesium, Phosphorus
Cashews	1 oz	157	9	5	12.4	0.9	Copper, Magnesium, Manganese
Pecans	1 oz	193	4	2.6	20.4	2.7	Manganese, Copper, Thiamine
Brazil Nuts	1 oz	186	3.4	4	18.8	2.1	Selenium, Copper, Magnesium
Macadamia Nuts	1 oz	204	3	2	21.5	2.4	Monounsaturated Fats, Thiamine, Copper
Hazelnuts	1 oz	176	5	4	17	2.7	Vitamin E, Copper, Manganese
Pistachios	1 oz	156	8	6	12.9	2.9	Vitamin B6, Copper, Manganese
Sesame Seeds	1 oz	160	7	4.8	13.6	3.3	Copper, Manganese, Magnesium
Hemp Seeds	1 oz	162	3	9.2	12.6	1.2	Calcium, Iron, Magnesium

Dark Chocolate (70-85%)	1 oz	170	12	2	12	3	Iron, Magnesium, Copper, Manganese
Olive Oil	1 tbsp	119	0	0	13.5	0	Vitamin E, Vitamin K, Antioxidants
Coconut Oil	1 tbsp	121	0	0	13.5	0	Lauric Acid, Medium-Chain Triglycerides, Antioxidants
Almonds	1 oz	164	6	6	14	3.5	Vitamin E, Magnesium, Riboflavin
Walnuts	1 oz	185	4	4	18.5	2	Omega-3 Fatty Acids, Vitamin E, Antioxidants
Chia Seeds	1 oz	138	12	4.7	8.7	9.8	Calcium, Iron, Magnesium
Flaxseeds	1 tbsp	37	1.6	1.3	3	1.9	Omega-3 Fatty Acids, Fiber, Vitamin B1
Sunflower Seeds	1 oz	164	6	5	14.2	2.4	Vitamin E, Copper, Magnesium

Pumpkin Seeds	1 oz	151	5	7	13	1.7	Magnesium, Phosphorus, Manganese
Peanut Butter	2 tbsp	188	6	8	16	2	Vitamin E, Niacin, Magnesium, Phosphorus
Cashews	1 oz	157	9	5	12.4	0.9	Copper, Magnesium, Manganese
Pecans	1 oz	193	4	2.6	20.4	2.7	Manganese, Copper, Thiamine
Brazil Nuts	1 oz	186	3.4	4	18.8	2.1	Selenium, Copper, Magnesium
Macadamia Nuts	1 oz	204	3	2	21.5	2.4	Monounsaturated Fats, Thiamine, Copper
Hazelnuts	1 oz	176	5	4	17	2.7	Vitamin E, Copper, Manganese
Pistachios	1 oz	156	8	6	12.9	2.9	Vitamin B6, Copper, Manganese

Sesame Seeds	1 oz	160	7	4.8	13.6	3.3	Copper, Manganese, Magnesium
Hemp Seeds	1 oz	162	3	9.2	12.6	1.2	Calcium, Iron, Magnesium
Dark Chocolate (70-85%)	1 oz	170	12	2	12	3	Iron, Magnesium, Copper, Manganese

Vegetables and Fruits: Vitamins, Minerals, and Fiber

Food Name	Portion Size	Calories (kcal)	Carbohydrates (g)	Protein (g)	Fat (g)	Fiber (g)	Vitamins & Minerals
Spinach	1 cup (30g)	7	1	0.9	0.1	0.7	Vitamin K, Vitamin A, Folate, Iron, Calcium, Magnesium, Potassium
Broccoli	1 cup (91g)	55	11	4.7	0.6	2.4	Vitamin C, Vitamin K, Folate, Vitamin A, Fiber, Calcium, Iron, Potassium
Kale	1 cup (21g)	33	6	2.9	0.5	1.3	Vitamin K, Vitamin A,

							Vitamin C, Folate, Calcium, Potassium, Manganese
Carrots	1 medium (61g)	25	6		0.6	0.1	1.7	Vitamin A, Vitamin K, Potassium, Vitamin C, Fiber
Bell Peppers (Red)	1 medium (119g)	37	9		1.4	0.2	3.1	Vitamin C, Vitamin A, Vitamin B6, Folate, Fiber, Potassium
Bell Peppers (Green)	1 medium (119g)	24	6		1.2	0.2	2.5	Vitamin C, Vitamin A, Vitamin K, Folate, Fiber, Potassium
Bell Peppers (Yellow)	1 medium (119g)	50	12		1.9	0.3	3.6	Vitamin C, Vitamin A, Vitamin B6, Folate, Fiber, Potassium
Tomatoes	1 medium (123g)	22	5		1.1	0.2	1.5	Vitamin C, Vitamin K, Folate,

						Potassium, Lycopene
Cucumber	1/2 cup (52g)	8	2	0.3	0	0.3	Vitamin K, Potassium, Vitamin C, Magnesium
Cauliflower	1 cup (100g)	25	5	1.9	0.1	2	Vitamin C, Vitamin K, Folate, Fiber, Choline, Potassium
Brussels Sprouts	1 cup (88g)	38	8	3.0	0.3	3.3	Vitamin K, Vitamin C, Folate, Vitamin A, Fiber, Potassium
Asparagus	1/2 cup (90g)	20	4	2.2	0.2	2	Vitamin K, Folate, Vitamin A, Vitamin C, Fiber, Potassium, Iron
Zucchini	1 medium (196g)	33	6	2.4	0.6	2	Vitamin C, Vitamin K, Folate, Fiber, Potassium, Manganese

Celery	1 stalk (40g)	6	1	0.3	0	0.6	Vitamin K, Folate, Vitamin A, Fiber, Potassium, Manganese
Green Beans	1/2 cup (100g)	31	7	1.8	0.2	2.7	Vitamin K, Vitamin C, Folate, Fiber, Manganese, Potassium
Eggplant	1 cup (82g)	20	5	0.8	0.2	2.5	Vitamin K, Folate, Fiber, Vitamin C, Potassium, Manganese
Beets	1 cup (136g)	58	13	2.2	0.2	3.8	Folate, Vitamin C, Iron, Magnesium, Potassium, Fiber
Cabbage	1 cup (89g)	22	5	1.1	0.1	2	Vitamin K, Vitamin C, Folate, Fiber, Potassium, Manganese
Onions	1 medium (110g)	44	10	1.2	0	1.9	Vitamin C, Folate, Vitamin B6, Potassium,

							Fiber, Manganese
Artichokes	1 medium (120g)	60	13	3.5	0.2	6.9	Folate, Vitamin K, Vitamin C, Fiber, Magnesium, Potassium
Squash (Butternut)	1 cup (205g)	63	16	1.4	0.1	2	Vitamin A, Vitamin C, Fiber, Potassium, Magnesium, Manganese
Squash (Acorn)	1 cup (205g)	115	29	1.4	0.3	9	Vitamin A, Vitamin C, Fiber, Potassium, Magnesium, Manganese
Mushrooms	1 cup (70g)	15	2	2.2	0.2	0.7	Vitamin D, Vitamin B6, Folate, Riboflavin, Niacin, Pantothenic Acid, Selenium

Sweet Potatoes	1 medium (130g)	103	24	2.3	0	3.8	Vitamin A, Vitamin C, Manganese, Fiber, Vitamin B6, Potassium, Magnesium
Garlic	1 clove (3g)	4	1	0.2	0	0.1	Manganese, Vitamin B6, Vitamin C, Selenium, Fiber
Ginger	1 tsp (2g)	2	0.5	0.1	0	0.1	Manganese, Copper, Vitamin B6, Magnesium, Iron, Potassium
Onions (Red)	1 medium (110g)	37	9	1.1	0	1.7	Vitamin C, Folate, Vitamin B6, Potassium, Fiber, Manganese
Beets	1 cup (136g)	58	13	2.2	0.2	3.8	Folate, Vitamin C, Iron, Magnesium, Potassium, Fiber
Cabbage	1 cup (89g)	22	5	1.1	0.1	2	Vitamin K, Vitamin C, Folate, Fiber,

						Potassium, Manganese
Onions	1 medium (110g)	44	10	1.2	0	1.9	Vitamin C, Folate, Vitamin B6, Potassium, Fiber, Manganese
Artichokes	1 medium (120g)	60	13	3.5	0.2	6.9	Folate, Vitamin K, Vitamin C, Fiber, Magnesium, Potassium
Squash (Butternut)	1 cup (205g)	63	16	1.4	0.1	2	Vitamin A, Vitamin C, Fiber, Potassium, Magnesium, Manganese
Squash (Acorn)	1 cup (205g)	115	29	1.4	0.3	9	Vitamin A, Vitamin C, Fiber, Potassium, Magnesium, Manganese
Mushrooms	1 cup (70g)	15	2	2.2	0.2	0.7	Vitamin D, Vitamin B6, Folate, Riboflavin,

						Niacin, Pantothenic Acid, Selenium
Sweet Potatoes	1 medium (130g)	103	24	2.3	0	3.8	Vitamin A, Vitamin C, Manganese, Fiber, Vitamin B6, Potassium, Magnesium
Garlic	1 clove (3g)	4	1	0.2	0	0.1	Manganese, Vitamin B6, Vitamin C, Selenium, Fiber
Ginger	1 tsp (2g)	2	0.5	0.1	0	0.1	Manganese, Copper, Vitamin B6, Magnesium, Iron, Potassium
Onions (Red)	1 medium (110g)	37	9	1.1	0	1.7	Vitamin C, Folate, Vitamin B6, Potassium, Fiber, Manganese

Dairy and Alternatives: Calcium and Protein Sources

Food Name	Portion Size	Calories (kcal)	Carbohydrates (g)	Protein (g)	Fat (g)	Fiber (g)	Calcium (mg)	Other Nutrients
Greek Yogurt	1 cup (245g)	150	8	22	4	0	240	Vitamin D, Probiotics
Cottage Cheese	1/2 cup (113g)	110	3	14	5	0	140	Vitamin B12, Selenium, Riboflavin, Phosphorus
Skim Milk	1 cup (245g)	83	12	8	0	0	300	Vitamin D, Vitamin A, Riboflavin, Phosphorus
Soy Milk	1 cup (243g)	131	8	7	8	1	300	Vitamin D, Vitamin B12, Riboflavin, Magnesium
Almond Milk	1 cup (240g)	60	8	1	2.5	1	450	Vitamin D, Vitamin E
Coconut Milk	1 cup (240g)	45	1	0	4	0	450	Medium-Chain Triglycerides, Vitamin D
Cashew Milk	1 cup (240g)	25	1	0	2.5	0	300	Vitamin D, Vitamin B12

Oat Milk	1 cup (240g)	130	24	4	2.5	2	350	Iron, Vitamin D, Riboflavin, Calcium, Vitamin B12
Hemp Milk	1 cup (240g)	70	1	3	6	0	300	Omega-3 Fatty Acids, Vitamin D
Rice Milk	1 cup (240g)	120	22	1	2.5	0	300	Vitamin D, Calcium, Iron, Vitamin B12
Greek Yogurt	1 cup (245g)	150	8	22	4	0	240	Vitamin D, Probiotics
Cottage Cheese	1/2 cup (113g)	110	3	14	5	0	140	Vitamin B12, Selenium, Riboflavin, Phosphorus
Skim Milk	1 cup (245g)	83	12	8	0	0	300	Vitamin D, Vitamin A, Riboflavin, Phosphorus
Soy Milk	1 cup (243g)	131	8	7	8	1	300	Vitamin D, Vitamin B12, Riboflavin, Magnesium

Almond Milk	1 cup (240g)	60	8	1	2.5	1	450	Vitamin D, Vitamin E
Coconut Milk	1 cup (240g)	45	1	0	4	0	450	Medium-Chain Triglycerides, Vitamin D
Cashew Milk	1 cup (240g)	25	1	0	2.5	0	300	Vitamin D, Vitamin B12
Oat Milk	1 cup (240g)	130	24	4	2.5	2	350	Iron, Vitamin D, Riboflavin, Calcium, Vitamin B12
Hemp Milk	1 cup (240g)	70	1	3	6	0	300	Omega-3 Fatty Acids, Vitamin D
Rice Milk	1 cup (240g)	120	22	1	2.5	0	300	Vitamin D, Calcium, Iron, Vitamin B12
Greek Yogurt	1 cup (245g)	150	8	22	4	0	240	Vitamin D, Probiotics
Cottage Cheese	1/2 cup (113g)	110	3	14	5	0	140	Vitamin B12, Selenium, Riboflavin, Phosphorus

Skim Milk	1 cup (245g)	83	12	8	0	0	300	Vitamin D, Vitamin A, Riboflavin, Phosphorus
Soy Milk	1 cup (243g)	131	8	7	8	1	300	Vitamin D, Vitamin B12, Riboflavin, Magnesium
Almond Milk	1 cup (240g)	60	8	1	2.5	1	450	Vitamin D, Vitamin E
Coconut Milk	1 cup (240g)	45	1	0	4	0	450	Medium-Chain Triglycerides, Vitamin D
Cashew Milk	1 cup (240g)	25	1	0	2.5	0	300	Vitamin D, Vitamin B12
Oat Milk	1 cup (240g)	130	24	4	2.5	2	350	Iron, Vitamin D, Riboflavin, Calcium, Vitamin B12
Hemp Milk	1 cup (240g)	70	1	3	6	0	300	Omega-3 Fatty Acids, Vitamin D
Rice Milk	1 cup (240g)	120	22	1	2.5	0	300	Vitamin D, Calcium,

								Iron, Vitamin B12

Beverages: Staying Hydrated

Food Name	Portion Size	Calories (kcal)	Carbohydrates (g)	Protein (g)	Fat (g)	Fiber (g)	Other Nutrients
Water	8 oz (240 ml)	0	0	0	0	0	Hydration
Herbal Tea	8 oz (240 ml)	0	0	0	0	0	Antioxidants
Green Tea	8 oz (240 ml)	2	0	0.5	0	0	Catechins, Caffeine
Black Tea	8 oz (240 ml)	2	0.5	0.2	0	0	Caffeine, Antioxidants
Chamomile Tea	8 oz (240 ml)	2	0.4	0	0	0	Antioxidants, Relaxation
Peppermint Tea	8 oz (240 ml)	2	0.5	0	0	0	Antioxidants, Digestive Aid

Lemon Water	8 oz (240 ml)	6	2	0	0	0	Vitamin C, Hydration
Cucumber Water	8 oz (240 ml)	0	0	0	0	0	Hydration, Refreshment
Coconut Water	8 oz (240 ml)	45	8	2	0	2	Electrolytes, Hydration
Electrolyte Drinks	8 oz (240 ml)	Varies	Varies	Varies	Varies	Varies	Electrolytes, Hydration
Sparkling Water	8 oz (240 ml)	0	0	0	0	0	Hydration, Carbonation
Fruit Infused Water	8 oz (240 ml)	0	0	0	0	0	Hydration, Natural Flavor
Almond Milk	8 oz (240 ml)	60	8	1	2.5	1	Calcium, Vitamin E
Soy Milk	8 oz (240 ml)	131	8	7	8	1	Protein, Calcium, Vitamin D

Oat Milk	8 oz (240 ml)	130	24	4	2.5	2	Fiber, Calcium, Vitamin D
Rice Milk	8 oz (240 ml)	120	22	1	2.5	0	Iron, Vitamin B12, Calcium
Cashew Milk	8 oz (240 ml)	25	1	0	2.5	0	Vitamin D, Calcium
Hemp Milk	8 oz (240 ml)	70	1	3	6	0	Omega-3 Fatty Acids, Protein
Fruit Juice	8 oz (240 ml)	Varies	Varies	Varies	Varies	Varies	Vitamins, Minerals
Vegetable Juice	8 oz (240 ml)	Varies	Varies	Varies	Varies	Varies	Vitamins, Minerals
Tomato Juice	8 oz (240 ml)	41	10	2	0.4	2	Vitamin C, Lycopene
Orange Juice	8 oz (240 ml)	110	26	2	0	0	Vitamin C, Calcium

Apple Juice	8 oz (240 ml)	114	28	0.5	0	0	Vitamin C, Potassium
Grape Juice	8 oz (240 ml)	152	36	1	0	0	Vitamin C, Resveratrol
Cranberry Juice	8 oz (240 ml)	116	31	0	0	0	Vitamin C, Antioxidants
Pineapple Juice	8 oz (240 ml)	132	33	0.5	0	0	Vitamin C, Bromelain
Lemonade	8 oz (240 ml)	99	26	0	0	0	Vitamin C, Hydration
Iced Tea	8 oz (240 ml)	4	1	0	0	0	Antioxidants, Hydration
Coffee	8 oz (240 ml)	2	0	0.3	0	0	Caffeine
Decaf Coffee	8 oz (240 ml)	2	0.5	0.1	0	0	Caffeine

Protein Shake	8 oz (240 ml)	Varies	Varies	Varies	Varies	Varies	Protein, Vitamins, Minerals
Smoothie	8 oz (240 ml)	Varies	Varies	Varies	Varies	Varies	Vitamins, Minerals, Fiber
Kombucha	8 oz (240 ml)	30	7	0	0	0	Probiotics, Antioxidants
Sports Drink	8 oz (240 ml)	80	21	0	0	0	Electrolytes, Hydration
Coconut Water	8 oz (240 ml)	45	8	2	0	2	Electrolytes, Hydration
Electrolyte Drinks	8 oz (240 ml)	Varies	Varies	Varies	Varies	Varies	Electrolytes, Hydration
Sparkling Water	8 oz (240 ml)	0	0	0	0	0	Hydration, Carbonation
Fruit Infused Water	8 oz (240 ml)	0	0	0	0	0	Hydration, Natural Flavor

These beverages offer a variety of options to help individuals stay hydrated while following the Metabolic Confusion Diet, providing essential nutrients and refreshing flavors without excessive sugars or additives.

Foods to Limit or Avoid

Limiting or avoiding certain foods is crucial for maintaining a healthy diet and achieving your wellness goals. In the context of the Metabolic Confusion Diet, it's important to understand which foods may hinder your progress and make informed choices accordingly.

- **Processed Foods:** These are foods that have undergone extensive processing and often contain high amounts of refined sugars, unhealthy fats, sodium, and artificial additives. Examples include sugary cereals, processed meats like bacon and sausage, packaged snacks, and pre-packaged meals. These ingredients can disrupt your metabolic health, leading to fluctuations in blood sugar levels, hormonal imbalances, and weight gain over time. To support your overall well-being, it's best to minimize or eliminate processed foods from your diet.

- **Added Sugars:** Excessive consumption of added sugars is associated with various health issues, including obesity, type 2 diabetes, cardiovascular disease, and metabolic syndrome. While natural sugars found in fruits and dairy are generally acceptable in moderation, added sugars in processed foods and beverages pose a significant risk to your metabolic health. Examples include table sugar, high-fructose corn syrup, and other sweeteners added to soft drinks, candies, baked goods, and condiments. To avoid these risks, it's advisable to check food labels carefully and choose products with minimal added sugars.

- **Trans Fats:** Trans fats, also known as partially hydrogenated oils, are artificial fats commonly found in fried foods, baked goods, margarine, and processed snacks. These fats have detrimental effects on cardiovascular health and metabolic function, increasing LDL (bad) cholesterol levels, reducing HDL (good) cholesterol levels, promoting inflammation, and insulin resistance. To support your metabolic health and reduce the risk of chronic diseases, it's best to avoid trans fats altogether and opt for healthier fat sources like avocados, nuts, seeds, and olive oil.

- **Refined Carbohydrates:** Refined carbohydrates lack fiber and essential nutrients due to processing, resulting in empty calories that can cause rapid spikes in blood sugar levels and contribute to insulin resistance. Examples include white bread, white rice, pasta, pastries, sugary cereals, and baked goods made with white flour. These foods can lead to energy crashes, increased hunger, and weight gain over time. Instead, prioritize whole, unprocessed carbohydrates like whole grains, fruits, vegetables, and legumes, which provide fiber, vitamins, minerals, and sustained energy.

- **Artificial Sweeteners:** Marketed as a healthier alternative to sugar, artificial sweeteners may have adverse effects on metabolic health. Research suggests that they can disrupt the gut microbiota, increase cravings for sweet foods, and interfere with insulin signaling, potentially leading to metabolic dysregulation and weight gain. While the long-term safety of artificial sweeteners is still debated, it's wise to consume them in moderation and opt for natural sweeteners like stevia, monk fruit, and honey when necessary.

CHAPTER 6

MEAL PLANNING AND PREPARATION

Setting Up Your Kitchen

Creating an environment that supports healthy eating is crucial for success on the Metabolic Confusion Diet. By organizing your kitchen thoughtfully, you can simplify meal preparation, minimize food waste, and make healthier choices more accessible. Here are some practical tips to set up your kitchen for success:

1. **Declutter:** Start by clearing out any items that may tempt you to veer off course from your dietary goals. Remove processed snacks, sugary treats, and unhealthy convenience foods that don't align with your wellness objectives. This decluttering process not only creates physical space but also fosters mental clarity and focus on your health journey.

2. **Stock Up Smartly:** Once you've decluttered, take stock of essential staples for a healthy diet. Whole grains, legumes, nuts, seeds, herbs, spices, healthy oils, and condiments form the foundation. Consider investing in diverse whole grains like brown rice, quinoa, oats, and whole wheat pasta, along with nuts, seeds, and plant-based proteins for added flavor and nutrition.

3. **Organize Your Pantry:** Arrange pantry items systematically to facilitate easy access and meal planning. Group similar items together, label containers for quick identification, and keep healthier options visible. Consider investing in storage containers to maximize shelf space and keep ingredients fresh.

4. **Functional Workspace:** Designate a clear workspace for meal preparation and cooking activities. Keep essential tools and utensils easily accessible, such as knives, cutting boards, and measuring cups. This organization streamlines meal prep and minimizes time spent searching for tools.

5. **Quality Cookware:** Invest in durable, non-toxic cookware like stainless steel or ceramic pots and pans. Versatile kitchen gadgets such as blenders and food processors can expand your culinary options and simplify meal prep.

6. **Green Corner:** Incorporating fresh herbs and greens into your kitchen not only adds flavor but also nutrition and visual appeal to your meals. Grow herbs indoors or install a wall planter for easy access to fresh ingredients.

7. **Food Safety:** Prioritize food safety to prevent illness and maintain ingredient freshness. Wash produce thoroughly, store perishables at the correct temperature, and clean kitchen surfaces regularly.

Shopping Tips for Healthy Eating

Navigating the grocery store can be overwhelming, but with a strategic approach, you can make informed choices that support your dietary goals. Here are some practical tips for healthy grocery shopping:

1. **Plan Ahead:** Plan your meals for the week and create a detailed shopping list. Incorporate a variety of nutrient-dense foods from all food groups to ensure balanced nutrition.

2. **Shop the Perimeter:** Focus on the outer aisles of the store where fresh produce, meats, dairy, and whole foods are typically located. This strategy prioritizes nutrient-rich options and avoids processed foods.

3. **Read Labels:** Scrutinize food labels for added sugars, unhealthy fats, and artificial additives. Opt for products with recognizable, whole-food ingredients and pay attention to serving sizes and nutrient content.

4. **Choose Whole Foods:** Prefer whole, minimally processed foods over refined options. Select whole grains, fresh or frozen fruits and vegetables, and lean proteins to maximize nutrition.

5. **Shop Seasonally:** Take advantage of seasonal produce for freshness and flavor. Seasonal fruits and vegetables are often more affordable and nutritious than out-of-season options.

6. **Portion Control:** Practice portion control to maintain a healthy balance of nutrients and energy intake. Use measuring tools to portion out servings and listen to your body's hunger and fullness cues.

7. **Stick to Budget:** Plan meals around affordable, nutrient-dense foods and look for sales and discounts. Consider buying in bulk or opting for generic brands to save money without sacrificing quality.

8. **Mindful Shopping:** Approach grocery shopping with mindfulness and intentionality. Avoid shopping when hungry and savor the experience of selecting fresh, wholesome foods that nourish your body and support your well-being.

Breakfast Recipes

Blueberry Almond Overnight Oats

Prep Time: 5 minutes

Cooking Time: 0 minutes

Serving Size: 1 bowl

Ingredients:

- 1/2 cup rolled oats

- 1/2 cup unsweetened almond milk

- 1/4 cup Greek yogurt

- 1/2 tbsp chia seeds

- 1/2 tbsp almond butter

- 1/2 cup fresh blueberries

- 1 tbsp honey or maple syrup (optional)

- Sliced almonds, for topping

Instructions:

1. In a bowl or jar, combine rolled oats, almond milk, Greek yogurt, chia seeds, and almond butter.

2. Stir well to mix all ingredients thoroughly.

3. Gently fold in fresh blueberries.

4. Cover and refrigerate overnight, or for at least 4 hours.

5. Before serving, drizzle with honey or maple syrup if desired and sprinkle with sliced almonds.

Nutritional Information (per serving):

- Calories: 320

- Protein: 13g

- Sodium: 92mg

- Potassium: 280mg

- Total Fat: 9g

- Saturated Fat: 1g

- Cholesterol: 3mg

- Carbohydrates: 52g

- Fiber: 9g

- Sugars: 15g

Spinach and Feta Egg Muffins

Prep Time: 10 minutes
Cooking Time: 20 minutes
Serving Size: 2 muffins

Ingredients:

- 6 large eggs

- 1/4 cup milk or unsweetened almond milk

- 1 cup fresh spinach, chopped

- 1/4 cup crumbled feta cheese

- 1/4 cup diced tomatoes

- Salt and pepper, to taste

- Cooking spray or olive oil, for greasing

Instructions:

1. Preheat oven to 350°F and grease a muffin tin with cooking spray or olive oil.

2. In a mixing bowl, whisk together eggs and milk until well combined.

3. Stir in chopped spinach, crumbled feta cheese, diced tomatoes, salt, and pepper.

4. Pour the egg mixture evenly into the prepared muffin tin, filling each cup about 2/3 full.

5. Bake in the preheated oven for 18-20 minutes or until the egg muffins are set and lightly golden on top.

6. Remove from the oven and allow to cool slightly before serving.

Nutritional Information (per serving):

- Calories: 155

- Protein: 12g

- Sodium: 298mg

- Potassium: 244mg

- Total Fat: 10g

- Saturated Fat: 4g

- Cholesterol: 311mg

- Carbohydrates: 3g

- Fiber: 1g

- Sugars: 2g

Quinoa Breakfast Bowl

Prep Time: 10 minutes

Cooking Time: 15 minutes

Serving Size: 1 bowl

Ingredients:

- 1/2 cup cooked quinoa

- 1/4 cup unsweetened almond milk

- 1/2 tsp ground cinnamon

- 1/4 tsp vanilla extract

- 1 tbsp honey or maple syrup

- 1/2 banana, sliced

- 1/4 cup mixed berries (strawberries, raspberries, blueberries)

- 1 tbsp chopped nuts (almonds, walnuts, pecans)

- 1 tbsp unsweetened shredded coconut (optional)

Instructions:

1. In a small saucepan, heat cooked quinoa with almond milk over medium heat.

2. Stir in ground cinnamon, vanilla extract, and honey or maple syrup until well combined.

3. Cook for 5-7 minutes, stirring occasionally, until heated through.

4. Transfer the quinoa mixture to a bowl and top with sliced banana, mixed berries, chopped nuts, and shredded coconut, if desired.

5. Serve warm and enjoy!

Nutritional Information (per serving):

- Calories: 290

- Protein: 7g

- Sodium: 48mg

- Potassium: 367mg

- Total Fat: 7g

- Saturated Fat: 1g

- Cholesterol: 0mg

- Carbohydrates: 52g

- Fiber: 7g

- Sugars: 19g

Avocado Toast with Poached Egg

Prep Time: 10 minutes

Cooking Time: 5 minutes

Serving Size: 1 slice of toast

Ingredients:

- 1 slice whole grain bread, toasted

- 1/2 ripe avocado, mashed

- 1 large egg

- Salt and pepper, to taste

- Red pepper flakes (optional)

- Chopped fresh herbs (cilantro, parsley, chives)

Instructions:

1. Toast a slice of whole-grain bread until golden brown.

2. Spread mashed avocado evenly on top of the toast.

3. Fill a small saucepan with water and bring to a gentle simmer.

4. Crack an egg into a small bowl, then carefully slide it into the simmering water.

5. Poach the egg for 3-4 minutes, until the whites are set but the yolk is still runny.

6. Using a slotted spoon, remove the poached egg from the water and place it on top of the avocado toast.

7. Season with salt, pepper, red pepper flakes, and chopped fresh herbs.

8. Serve immediately and enjoy!

Nutritional Information (per serving):

- Calories: 220

- Protein: 11g

- Sodium: 220mg

- Potassium: 430mg

- Total Fat: 12g

- Saturated Fat: 2g

- Cholesterol: 186mg

- Carbohydrates: 18g

- Fiber: 6g

- Sugars: 1g

Greek Yogurt Parfait

Prep Time: 5 minutes

Cooking Time: 0 minutes

Serving Size: 1 parfait

Ingredients:

- 1/2 cup plain Greek yogurt

- 1/4 cup granola (choose a low-sugar option)

- 1/2 cup mixed berries (strawberries, blueberries, raspberries)

- 1 tbsp honey or maple syrup (optional)

- 1 tbsp sliced almonds or chopped walnuts

Instructions:

1. In a glass or bowl, layer half of the Greek yogurt.

2. Add half of the granola on top of the yogurt layer.

3. Layer half of the mixed berries over the granola.

4. Repeat the layers with the remaining Greek yogurt, granola, and mixed berries.

5. Drizzle with honey or maple syrup if desired and sprinkle with sliced almonds or chopped walnuts.

6. Serve immediately and enjoy!

Nutritional Information (per serving):

- Calories: 280

- Protein: 15g

- Sodium: 80mg

- Potassium: 240mg

- Total Fat: 7g

- Saturated Fat: 1g

- Cholesterol: 0mg

- Carbohydrates: 45g

- Fiber: 6g

- Sugars: 22g

Sweet Potato Breakfast Hash

Prep Time: 10 minutes

Cooking Time: 20 minutes

Serving Size: 1 plate

Ingredients:

- 1 small sweet potato, peeled and diced

- 1/4 cup diced red bell pepper

- 1/4 cup diced onion

- 1/4 cup diced zucchini

- 2 large eggs

- 1 tbsp olive oil or avocado oil

- Salt and pepper, to taste

- Fresh herbs (parsley, chives) for garnish

Instructions:

1. Heat olive oil or avocado oil in a skillet over medium heat.

2. Add diced sweet potato to the skillet and cook for 5-7 minutes, until slightly softened.

3. Add diced red bell pepper, onion, and zucchini to the skillet and continue cooking for another 5-7 minutes, until vegetables are tender.

4. Create two wells in the vegetable mixture and crack an egg into each well.

5. Season with salt and pepper to taste.

6. Cover the skillet and cook for 5-7 minutes, until the egg whites are set but the yolks are still runny.

7. Remove from heat and garnish with fresh herbs.

8. Serve hot and enjoy!

Nutritional Information (per serving):

- Calories: 330
- Protein: 11g
- Sodium: 130mg
- Potassium: 950mg
- Total Fat: 15g
- Saturated Fat: 3g
- Cholesterol: 186mg
- Carbohydrates: 40g
- Fiber: 7g
- Sugars: 9g

Whole Grain Pancakes

Prep Time: 10 minutes

Cooking Time: 10 minutes

Serving Size: 2 pancakes

Ingredients:

- 1/2 cup whole wheat flour
- 1/4 cup oat flour
- 1 tbsp ground flaxseed
- 1 tsp baking powder
- 1/2 tsp ground cinnamon
- 1/2 cup unsweetened almond milk
- 1 large egg

- 1 tbsp honey or maple syrup

- 1/2 tsp vanilla extract

- Cooking spray or olive oil, for greasing

- Fresh fruit (berries, sliced banana) for topping

Instructions:

1. In a mixing bowl, whisk together whole wheat flour, oat flour, ground flaxseed, baking powder, and ground cinnamon.

2. In a separate bowl, whisk together almond milk, egg, honey or maple syrup, and vanilla extract.

3. Pour the wet ingredients into the dry ingredients and stir until just combined. Do not overmix.

4. Heat a non-stick skillet or griddle over medium heat and lightly coat with cooking spray or olive oil.

5. Pour 1/4 cup of pancake batter onto the skillet for each pancake.

6. Cook for 2-3 minutes on each side, until golden brown and cooked through.

7. Serve warm with fresh fruit toppings and a drizzle of honey or maple syrup if desired.

8. Enjoy your nutritious and delicious pancakes!

Nutritional Information (per serving):

- Calories: 280

- Protein: 10g

- Sodium: 260mg

- Potassium: 170mg

- Total Fat: 7g

- Saturated Fat: 1g

- Cholesterol: 93mg

- Carbohydrates: 45g

- Fiber: 5g

- Sugars: 12g

Spinach and Mushroom Omelette

Prep Time: 10 minutes

Cooking Time: 10 minutes

Serving Size: 1 omelette

Ingredients:

- 2 large eggs

- 1/4 cup sliced mushrooms

- 1/2 cup fresh spinach leaves

- 1/4 cup diced onion

- 1/4 cup diced tomato

- 1 tbsp olive oil

- Salt and pepper, to taste

- 2 tbsp shredded cheese (optional)

Instructions:

1. In a small bowl, whisk the eggs until well beaten. Set aside.

2. Heat olive oil in a non-stick skillet over medium heat.

3. Add sliced mushrooms, diced onion, and diced tomato to the skillet. Cook until vegetables are softened, about 3-4 minutes.

4. Add fresh spinach leaves to the skillet and cook until wilted, about 1-2 minutes.

5. Pour the beaten eggs over the cooked vegetables in the skillet.

6. Allow the eggs to set around the edges, then gently lift the edges of the omelet and tilt the skillet to let the uncooked eggs flow underneath.

7. Once the eggs are almost set, sprinkle shredded cheese over one-half of the omelet if desired.

8. Fold the omelet in half and cook for another 1-2 minutes, until the cheese is melted and the eggs are cooked through.

9. Season with salt and pepper to taste.

10. Slide the omelet onto a plate and serve hot.

Nutritional Information (per serving):

- Calories: 280
- Protein: 17g
- Sodium: 340mg
- Potassium: 480mg
- Total Fat: 20g
- Saturated Fat: 6g
- Cholesterol: 380mg
- Carbohydrates: 7g
- Fiber: 2g
- Sugars: 3g

Avocado Toast with Poached Egg

Prep Time: 5 minutes

Cooking Time: 5 minutes

Serving Size: 1 toast

Ingredients:

- 1 slice whole grain bread

- 1/2 ripe avocado, mashed

- 1 large egg

- Salt and pepper, to taste

- Red pepper flakes (optional)

- Fresh herbs (cilantro, parsley) for garnish

Instructions:

1. Toast the whole-grain bread until golden brown.

2. Spread the mashed avocado evenly on the toasted bread slice.

3. Bring a pot of water to a gentle simmer over medium heat. Add a splash of vinegar to the water.

4. Crack the egg into a small bowl.

5. Using a spoon, create a whirlpool in the simmering water and carefully slide the egg into the center of the whirlpool.

6. Poach the egg for 3-4 minutes, until the egg white is set but the yolk is still runny.

7. Remove the poached egg from the water using a slotted spoon and place it on top of the avocado toast.

8. Season with salt, pepper, and red pepper flakes if desired.

9. Garnish with fresh herbs and serve immediately.

Nutritional Information (per serving):

- Calories: 270

- Protein: 11g

- Sodium: 210mg

- Potassium: 530mg

- Total Fat: 17g

- Saturated Fat: 3g

- Cholesterol: 185mg

- Carbohydrates: 20g

- Fiber: 8g

- Sugars: 2g

Quinoa Breakfast Bowl

Prep Time: 10 minutes

Cooking Time: 15 minutes

Serving Size: 1 bowl

Ingredients:

- 1/2 cup cooked quinoa

- 1/4 cup unsweetened almond milk

- 1/2 tsp ground cinnamon

- 1/2 cup mixed berries (strawberries, blueberries, raspberries)

- 1 tbsp almond butter

- 1 tbsp chopped nuts (almonds, walnuts, pecans)

- 1 tsp honey or maple syrup (optional)

- Fresh mint leaves for garnish

Instructions:

1. In a small saucepan, heat cooked quinoa and almond milk over medium heat.

2. Stir in ground cinnamon and cook until heated through, about 2-3 minutes.

3. Transfer the quinoa mixture to a bowl.

4. Top with mixed berries, almond butter, and chopped nuts.

5. Drizzle with honey or maple syrup if desired.

6. Garnish with fresh mint leaves.

7. Serve warm and enjoy!

Nutritional Information (per serving):

- Calories: 320

- Protein: 10g

- Sodium: 60mg

- Potassium: 310mg

- Total Fat: 14g

- Saturated Fat: 1g

- Cholesterol: 0mg

- Carbohydrates: 40g

- Fiber: 7g

- Sugars: 9g

Lunch Recipes

Grilled Chicken Salad with Balsamic Vinaigrette

Prep Time: 15 minutes

Cooking Time: 15 minutes

Serving Size: 1 salad

Ingredients:

- 4 oz boneless, skinless chicken breast

- Salt and pepper, to taste

- 2 cups mixed salad greens (spinach, arugula, romaine)

- 1/4 cup cherry tomatoes, halved

- 1/4 cup cucumber, sliced

- 1/4 cup bell pepper, diced

- 1/4 cup red onion, thinly sliced

- 1 tbsp olive oil

- 1 tbsp balsamic vinegar

- 1/2 tsp Dijon mustard

- 1/2 tsp honey (optional)

Instructions:

1. Season the chicken breast with salt and pepper.

2. Heat a grill or grill pan over medium-high heat. Grill the chicken breast for 6-8 minutes per side, or until cooked through and no longer pink in the center.

3. In a small bowl, whisk together olive oil, balsamic vinegar, Dijon mustard, and honey (if using) to make the vinaigrette.

4. In a large bowl, combine mixed salad greens, cherry tomatoes, cucumber, bell pepper, and red onion.

5. Slice the grilled chicken breast and add it to the salad.

6. Drizzle the balsamic vinaigrette over the salad and toss gently to coat.

7. Serve immediately.

Nutritional Information (per serving):

- Calories: 280

- Protein: 30g

- Sodium: 380mg

- Potassium: 750mg

- Total Fat: 12g

- Saturated Fat: 2g

- Cholesterol: 80mg

- Carbohydrates: 12g

- Fiber: 3g

- Sugars: 7g

Turkey and Avocado Wrap

Prep Time: 10 minutes

Cooking Time: 0 minutes

Serving Size: 1 wrap

Ingredients:

- 1 whole wheat tortilla

- 3 oz sliced turkey breast

- 1/4 avocado, sliced

- 1/4 cup mixed salad greens

- 2 slices tomato

- 1 tbsp hummus

- Salt and pepper, to taste

Instructions:

1. Lay the whole wheat tortilla flat on a clean surface.

2. Spread hummus evenly over the tortilla.

3. Layer sliced turkey breast, avocado slices, mixed salad greens, and tomato slices on top of
   the hummus.

4. Season with salt and pepper to taste.

5. Roll up the tortilla tightly, folding in the sides as you go.

6. Slice the wrap in half diagonally.

7. Serve immediately or wrap in parchment paper for later.

Nutritional Information (per serving):

- Calories: 320

- Protein: 25g

- Sodium: 590mg

- Potassium: 570mg

- Total Fat: 14g

- Saturated Fat: 3g

- Cholesterol: 40mg

- Carbohydrates: 28g

- Fiber: 7g

- Sugars: 2g

Salmon and Quinoa Bowl

Prep Time: 10 minutes
Cooking Time: 20 minutes
Serving Size: 1 bowl

Ingredients:

- 4 oz salmon fillet

- Salt and pepper, to taste

- 1/2 cup cooked quinoa

- 1/4 cup steamed broccoli florets

- 1/4 cup shredded carrots

- 1/4 cup diced cucumber

- 2 tbsp sliced almonds

- 1 tbsp chopped fresh parsley

- 1 tbsp lemon juice

- 1 tsp olive oil

Instructions:

1. Preheat the oven to 400°F. Season the salmon fillet with salt, pepper, and a squeeze of lemon juice.

2. Place the salmon fillet on a baking sheet lined with parchment paper. Bake for 12-15 minutes, or until the salmon is cooked through and flakes easily with a fork.

3. In a bowl, combine cooked quinoa, steamed broccoli florets, shredded carrots, diced cucumber, sliced almonds, chopped fresh parsley, lemon juice, and olive oil. Mix well.

4. Transfer the quinoa mixture to a serving bowl.

5. Top with the baked salmon fillet.

6. Serve hot or cold.

Nutritional Information (per serving):

- Calories: 380

- Protein: 30g

- Sodium: 300mg

- Potassium: 850mg

- Total Fat: 18g

- Saturated Fat: 2.5g

- Cholesterol: 65mg

- Carbohydrates: 24g

- Fiber: 5g

- Sugars: 2g

Quinoa and Black Bean Salad

Prep Time: 15 minutes

Cooking Time: 15 minutes

Serving Size: 1 bowl

Ingredients:

- 1/2 cup quinoa, rinsed

- 1 cup water or vegetable broth

- 1/2 cup black beans, cooked

- 1/4 cup corn kernels, cooked

- 1/4 cup cherry tomatoes, halved

- 1/4 cup red bell pepper, diced

- 2 tbsp red onion, finely chopped

- 2 tbsp fresh cilantro, chopped

- 1 tbsp lime juice

- 1 tbsp olive oil

- Salt and pepper, to taste

- Optional toppings: avocado slices, diced jalapeño, shredded cheese

Instructions:

1. In a saucepan, combine quinoa and water or vegetable broth. Bring to a boil, then reduce heat to low, cover, and simmer for 15 minutes, or until quinoa is cooked and liquid is absorbed. Fluff quinoa with a fork and let cool.

2. In a large bowl, combine cooked quinoa, black beans, corn kernels, cherry tomatoes, red bell pepper, red onion, and cilantro.

3. In a small bowl, whisk together lime juice, olive oil, salt, and pepper to make the dressing.

4. Pour the dressing over the quinoa mixture and toss gently to combine.

5. Taste and adjust seasoning as needed.

6. Serve the salad at room temperature or chilled, topped with optional toppings if desired.

Nutritional Information (per serving):

- Calories: 280

- Protein: 10g

- Sodium: 150mg

- Potassium: 400mg

- Total Fat: 8g

- Saturated Fat: 1g

- Cholesterol: 0mg

- Carbohydrates: 45g

- Fiber: 9g

- Sugars: 3g

Grilled Vegetable Quesadilla

Prep Time: 20 minutes

Cooking Time: 10 minutes

Serving Size: 1 quesadilla

Ingredients:

- 2 large whole wheat tortillas

- 1/2 cup black beans, cooked and mashed

- 1/2 cup mixed grilled vegetables (bell peppers, zucchini, onion, mushrooms), sliced

- 1/4 cup shredded cheese (cheddar, Monterey Jack, or a blend)

- 2 tbsp salsa

- 2 tbsp plain Greek yogurt or sour cream (optional)

- Cooking spray or olive oil, for grilling

Instructions:

1. Preheat a grill pan or skillet over medium heat.

2. Lay one tortilla flat on a clean surface. Spread mashed black beans evenly over the tortilla.

3. Arrange grilled vegetables on top of the black beans, then sprinkle shredded cheese over the vegetables.

4. Place the second tortilla on top to create a quesadilla.

5. Lightly coat both sides of the quesadilla with cooking spray or brush with olive oil.

6. Carefully transfer the quesadilla to the preheated grill pan or skillet.

7. Cook for 3-4 minutes on each side, or until tortillas are golden brown and crispy, and cheese is melted.

8. Remove the quesadilla from the grill and let it cool for a minute before slicing it into wedges.

9. Serve hot, with salsa and Greek yogurt or sour cream on the side for dipping, if desired.

Nutritional Information (per serving):

- Calories: 320

- Protein: 15g

- Sodium: 580mg

- Potassium: 330mg

- Total Fat: 12g

- Saturated Fat: 4g

- Cholesterol: 20mg

- Carbohydrates: 40g

- Fiber: 8g

- Sugars: 3g

Egg and Veggie Stir-Fry

Prep Time: 10 minutes

Cooking Time: 10 minutes

Serving Size: 1 serving

Ingredients:

- 2 large eggs

- 1 cup mixed vegetables (bell peppers, broccoli, snap peas, carrots), sliced

- 1/4 cup onion, thinly sliced

- 1 clove garlic, minced

- 1 tbsp low-sodium soy sauce or tamari

- 1/2 tsp sesame oil

- 1/2 tsp ginger, grated

- 1/4 tsp red pepper flakes (optional)
- 1 tbsp olive oil or cooking oil
- Salt and pepper, to taste
- Cooked brown rice or quinoa, for serving

Instructions:

1. Heat olive oil or cooking oil in a large skillet or wok over medium-high heat.
2. Add sliced onion and minced garlic to the skillet and cook for 1-2 minutes, until fragrant.
3. Add mixed vegetables to the skillet and stir-fry for 3-4 minutes, until vegetables are tender-crisp.
4. In a small bowl, whisk together eggs, soy sauce or tamari, sesame oil, grated ginger, and red pepper flakes (if using).
5. Push the vegetables to one side of the skillet and pour the egg mixture into the space.
6. Allow the eggs to cook undisturbed for a few seconds, then gently scramble until fully cooked.
7. Once the eggs are cooked, stir them into the vegetable mixture.
8. Season with salt and pepper to taste.
9. Serve the egg and veggie stir-fry hot cooked brown rice or quinoa.

Nutritional Information (per serving):

- Calories: 280
- Protein: 14g
- Sodium: 520mg
- Potassium: 350mg
- Total Fat: 16g
- Saturated Fat: 3.5g

- Cholesterol: 195mg

- Carbohydrates: 20g

- Fiber: 4g

- Sugars: 4g

Salmon Avocado Salad

Prep Time: 15 minutes

Cooking Time: 10 minutes

Serving Size: 1 salad

Ingredients:

- 4 oz salmon fillet

- Salt and pepper, to taste

- 2 cups mixed salad greens (spinach, arugula, kale)

- 1/2 avocado, sliced

- 1/4 cup cherry tomatoes, halved

- 1/4 cup cucumber, sliced

- 1/4 cup red onion, thinly sliced

- 1 tbsp olive oil

- 1 tbsp lemon juice

- 1 tsp Dijon mustard

- 1/2 tsp honey or maple syrup (optional)

Instructions:

1. Season the salmon fillet with salt and pepper to taste.

2. Heat olive oil in a skillet over medium heat. Add the salmon fillet to the skillet and cook for 3-4 minutes on each side, or until cooked through and flaky.

3. Remove the salmon from the skillet and let it cool slightly. Flake the salmon into bite-sized pieces.

4. In a large bowl, combine mixed salad greens, sliced avocado, cherry tomatoes, cucumber, and red onion.

5. In a small bowl, whisk together olive oil, lemon juice, Dijon mustard, honey or maple syrup (if using), salt, and pepper to make the dressing.

6. Pour the dressing over the salad and toss gently to coat.

7. Divide the salad onto serving plates and top with flaked salmon.

8. Serve the salmon avocado salad immediately.

Nutritional Information (per serving):

- Calories: 350

- Protein: 20g

- Sodium: 280mg

- Potassium: 860mg

- Total Fat: 24g

- Saturated Fat: 3.5g

- Cholesterol: 55mg

- Carbohydrates: 15g

- Fiber: 7g

- Sugars: 5g

Turkey and Vegetable Wrap

Prep Time: 10 minutes

Cooking Time: 10 minutes

Serving Size: 1 wrap

Ingredients:

- 1 whole wheat or spinach tortilla

- 2 oz cooked turkey breast, sliced

- 1/4 cup hummus

- 1/4 cup mixed salad greens (spinach, lettuce, arugula)

- 1/4 cup cucumber, thinly sliced

- 1/4 cup bell peppers (red, yellow, or green), thinly sliced

- 1/4 cup shredded carrots

- 1 tbsp feta cheese, crumbled

- Salt and pepper, to taste

Instructions:

1. Lay the tortilla flat on a clean surface.

2. Spread hummus evenly over the tortilla.

3. Layer sliced turkey breast, mixed salad greens, cucumber, bell peppers, shredded carrots, and crumbled feta cheese on top of the hummus.

4. Season with salt and pepper to taste.

5. Fold the sides of the tortilla inward, then roll it up tightly from the bottom to form a wrap.

6. Slice the wrap in half diagonally.

7. Serve the turkey and vegetable wrap immediately or wrap it in foil for later.

Nutritional Information (per serving):

- Calories: 280

- Protein: 20g

- Sodium: 620mg

- Potassium: 320mg

- Total Fat: 10g

- Saturated Fat: 2.5g

- Cholesterol: 30mg

- Carbohydrates: 25g

- Fiber: 6g

- Sugars: 3g

Greek Chicken Salad

Prep Time: 20 minutes

Cooking Time: 15 minutes

Serving Size: 1 salad

Ingredients:

- 4 oz grilled chicken breast, sliced

- Salt and pepper, to taste

- 2 cups mixed salad greens (romaine, spinach, kale)

- 1/4 cup cucumber, diced

- 1/4 cup cherry tomatoes, halved

- 1/4 cup red onion, thinly sliced

- 2 tbsp Kalamata olives, pitted and sliced

- 2 tbsp crumbled feta cheese

- 1 tbsp olive oil

- 1 tbsp lemon juice

- 1 tsp dried oregano

- 1/2 tsp garlic powder

Instructions:

1. Season the grilled chicken breast with salt, pepper, dried oregano, and garlic powder to taste.

2. In a large bowl, combine mixed salad greens, diced cucumber, cherry tomatoes, red onion, Kalamata olives, and crumbled feta cheese.

3. In a small bowl, whisk together olive oil and lemon juice to make the dressing.

4. Pour the dressing over the salad and toss gently to coat.

5. Divide the salad onto serving plates and top with sliced grilled chicken breast.

6. Serve the Greek chicken salad immediately.

Nutritional Information (per serving):

- Calories: 320

- Protein: 30g

- Sodium: 530mg

- Potassium: 770mg

- Total Fat: 15g

- Saturated Fat: 4g

- Cholesterol: 85mg

- Carbohydrates: 15g

- Fiber: 4g

- Sugars: 6g

Quinoa Salad with Chickpeas and Avocado

Prep Time: 15 minutes

Cooking Time: 15 minutes

Serving Size: 1 salad

Ingredients:

- 1/2 cup quinoa, rinsed

- 1 cup water or vegetable broth

- Salt, to taste

- 1/2 cup canned chickpeas, drained and rinsed

- 1/2 avocado, diced

- 1/4 cup cherry tomatoes, halved

- 1/4 cup cucumber, diced

- 2 tbsp red onion, finely chopped

- 2 tbsp fresh cilantro or parsley, chopped

- 1 tbsp olive oil

- 1 tbsp lemon juice

- 1/2 tsp cumin

- 1/4 tsp paprika

- 1/4 tsp garlic powder

- Salt and pepper, to taste

Instructions:

1. In a small saucepan, combine quinoa and water or vegetable broth. Bring to a boil, then reduce heat to low, cover, and simmer for 12-15 minutes, or until quinoa is cooked and liquid is absorbed. Fluff quinoa with a fork and let it cool slightly.

2. In a large bowl, combine cooked quinoa, chickpeas, diced avocado, cherry tomatoes, cucumber, red onion, and chopped cilantro or parsley.

3. In a small bowl, whisk together olive oil, lemon juice, cumin, paprika, garlic powder, salt, and pepper to make the dressing.

4. Pour the dressing over the quinoa salad and toss gently to coat.

5. Divide the salad onto serving plates and serve immediately, or store it in an airtight container in the refrigerator for later.

Nutritional Information (per serving):

- Calories: 320

- Protein: 10g

- Sodium: 230mg

- Potassium: 560mg

- Total Fat: 15g

- Saturated Fat: 2g

- Cholesterol: 0mg

- Carbohydrates: 40g

- Fiber: 8g

- Sugars: 2g

Dinner Recipes

Grilled Lemon Herb Chicken

Prep Time: 20 minutes

Marinating Time: 1 hour

Cooking Time: 15 minutes

Serving Size: 1 chicken breast

Ingredients:

- 2 boneless, skinless chicken breasts

- 2 tbsp olive oil

- Zest and juice of 1 lemon

- 2 cloves garlic, minced

- 1 tbsp fresh rosemary, chopped

- 1 tbsp fresh thyme leaves

- Salt and pepper, to taste

Instructions:

1. In a small bowl, whisk together olive oil, lemon zest, lemon juice, minced garlic, chopped rosemary, chopped thyme, salt, and pepper to create the marinade.

2. Place chicken breasts in a shallow dish or resealable plastic bag and pour the marinade over them. Ensure the chicken is evenly coated. Cover or seal and refrigerate for at least 1 hour, or overnight for best results.

3. Preheat the grill to medium-high heat. Remove chicken from marinade and discard excess marinade.

4. Grill chicken breasts for 6-7 minutes per side, or until cooked through and internal temperature reaches 165°F (75°C). Cooking time may vary depending on the thickness of the chicken breasts.

5. Remove chicken from the grill and let it rest for a few minutes before serving.

6. Serve grilled lemon herb chicken with your choice of side dishes, such as roasted vegetables, quinoa, or a green salad.

Nutritional Information (per serving):

- Calories: 280

- Protein: 26g

- Sodium: 120mg

- Potassium: 400mg

- Total Fat: 15g

- Saturated Fat: 2.5g

- Cholesterol: 70mg

- Carbohydrates: 3g

- Fiber: 1g

- Sugars: 0g

Baked Salmon with Asparagus

Prep Time: 10 minutes

Cooking Time: 15 minutes

Serving Size: 1 fillet

Ingredients:

- 2 salmon fillets

- 1 bunch asparagus, trimmed

- 2 tbsp olive oil

- 2 cloves garlic, minced

- 1 lemon, sliced

- Salt and pepper, to taste

- Fresh dill, for garnish

Instructions:

1. Preheat oven to 400°F (200°C). Line a baking sheet with parchment paper or aluminum foil.

2. Place salmon fillets on one side of the baking sheet and arrange asparagus spears on the other side.

3. Drizzle olive oil over salmon and asparagus. Sprinkle minced garlic evenly over both. Season with salt and pepper to taste.

4. Place lemon slices on top of the salmon fillets.

5. Bake in the preheated oven for 12-15 minutes, or until salmon is cooked through and flakes easily with a fork.

6. Remove from the oven and garnish with fresh dill before serving.

7. Serve baked salmon with asparagus alongside a side of brown rice or quinoa, if desired.

Nutritional Information (per serving):

- Calories: 320

- Protein: 30g

- Sodium: 120mg

- Potassium: 800mg

- Total Fat: 18g

- Saturated Fat: 2.5g

- Cholesterol: 80mg

- Carbohydrates: 8g

- Fiber: 4g

- Sugars: 2g

Stuffed Bell Peppers with Quinoa and Black Beans

Prep Time: 20 minutes

Cooking Time: 40 minutes

Serving Size: 1 stuffed pepper

Ingredients:

- 4 bell peppers, any color

- 1 cup quinoa, rinsed

- 2 cups vegetable broth

- 1 can (15 oz) black beans, drained and rinsed

- 1 cup corn kernels (fresh, frozen, or canned)

- 1 cup cherry tomatoes, halved

- 1/2 cup red onion, finely chopped

- 2 cloves garlic, minced

- 1 tsp ground cumin

- 1 tsp chili powder

- Salt and pepper, to taste

- 1/2 cup shredded cheddar cheese (optional)

- Fresh cilantro, for garnish

Instructions:

1. Preheat oven to 375°F (190°C). Slice the tops off the bell peppers and remove the seeds and membranes. Place the peppers upright in a baking dish.

2. In a medium saucepan, combine quinoa and vegetable broth. Bring to a boil, then reduce heat to low, cover, and simmer for 15-20 minutes, or until quinoa is cooked and liquid is absorbed.

3. In a large mixing bowl, combine cooked quinoa, black beans, corn kernels, cherry tomatoes, red onion, minced garlic, ground cumin, chili powder, salt, and pepper. Stir until well combined.

4. Spoon the quinoa mixture into each bell pepper until they are filled to the top. If using shredded cheese, sprinkle it over the top of each stuffed pepper.

5. Cover the baking dish with aluminum foil and bake in the preheated oven for 25-30 minutes, or until the peppers are tender.

6. Remove the foil and bake for an additional 5-10 minutes, or until the cheese is melted and bubbly.

7. Remove from the oven and let the stuffed peppers cool slightly before serving.

8. Garnish with fresh cilantro before serving, if desired.

Nutritional Information (per serving):

- Calories: 320

- Protein: 12g

- Sodium: 450mg

- Potassium: 750mg

- Total Fat: 5g

- Saturated Fat: 2g

- Cholesterol: 5mg

- Carbohydrates: 60g

- Fiber: 10g

- Sugars: 8g

Grilled Lemon Garlic Shrimp Skewers

Prep Time: 15 minutes

Marinating Time: 30 minutes

Cooking Time: 6 minutes

Serving Size: 2 skewers

Ingredients:

- 1 lb large shrimp, peeled and deveined

- 2 cloves garlic, minced

- Zest and juice of 1 lemon

- 2 tbsp olive oil

- 1 tsp dried oregano

- Salt and pepper, to taste

- Wooden or metal skewers

Instructions:

1. If using wooden skewers, soak them in water for at least 30 minutes to prevent burning.

2. In a bowl, whisk together minced garlic, lemon zest, lemon juice, olive oil, dried oregano, salt, and pepper to create the marinade.

3. Add shrimp to the marinade and toss to coat evenly. Cover and refrigerate for at least 30 minutes to allow the flavors to meld.

4. Preheat the grill to medium-high heat. Thread marinated shrimp onto skewers, dividing them evenly.

5. Grill shrimp skewers for 2-3 minutes per side, or until shrimp are pink and opaque.

6. Remove from the grill and serve immediately with your choice of side dishes, such as grilled vegetables, rice, or a salad.

Nutritional Information (per serving):

- Calories: 180

- Protein: 25g

- Sodium: 200mg

- Potassium: 180mg

- Total Fat: 7g

- Saturated Fat: 1g

- Cholesterol: 220mg

- Carbohydrates: 2g

- Fiber: 0g

- Sugars: 0g

Turkey and Vegetable Stir-Fry

Prep Time: 15 minutes
Cooking Time: 15 minutes
Serving Size: 1 cup

Ingredients:

- 1 lb turkey breast, thinly sliced

- 2 tbsp soy sauce (or tamari for gluten-free)

- 1 tbsp rice vinegar

- 1 tbsp honey or maple syrup

- 2 tbsp olive oil

- 2 cloves garlic, minced

- 1-inch piece ginger, grated

- 1 red bell pepper, thinly sliced

- 1 yellow bell pepper, thinly sliced

- 1 cup snap peas

- 1 cup broccoli florets

- Cooked brown rice or quinoa, for serving

- Sesame seeds, for garnish (optional)

- Sliced green onions, for garnish (optional)

Instructions:

1. In a small bowl, whisk together soy sauce, rice vinegar, and honey (or maple syrup) to create the sauce. Set aside.

2. Heat olive oil in a large skillet or wok over medium-high heat. Add minced garlic and grated ginger, and sauté for 1-2 minutes until fragrant.

3. Add sliced turkey breast to the skillet and stir-fry for 3-4 minutes until cooked through.

4. Add sliced bell peppers, snap peas, and broccoli florets to the skillet. Stir-fry for an additional 3-4 minutes until vegetables are tender-crisp.

5. Pour the prepared sauce over the turkey and vegetables in the skillet. Stir well to coat everything evenly.

6. Cook for 1-2 minutes, stirring occasionally, until the sauce thickens slightly and coats the turkey and vegetables.

7. Remove from heat and serve immediately over cooked brown rice or quinoa.

8. Garnish with sesame seeds and sliced green onions, if desired.

Nutritional Information (per serving):

- Calories: 250

- Protein: 25g

- Sodium: 600mg

- Potassium: 400mg

- Total Fat: 9g

- Saturated Fat: 1.5g

- Cholesterol: 50mg

- Carbohydrates: 15g

- Fiber: 3g

- Sugars: 6g

Salmon with Roasted Vegetables

Prep Time: 15 minutes

Cooking Time: 20 minutes

Serving Size: 1 fillet

Ingredients:

- 2 salmon fillets

- 2 tbsp olive oil, divided

- 1 tsp paprika

- 1 tsp garlic powder

- Salt and pepper, to taste

- 1 cup cherry tomatoes

- 1 bell pepper, sliced

- 1 zucchini, sliced

- 1 red onion, sliced

- Fresh parsley, chopped, for garnish (optional)

- Lemon wedges, for serving

Instructions:

1. Preheat oven to 400°F (200°C). Line a baking sheet with parchment paper.

2. Place salmon fillets on the prepared baking sheet. Drizzle with 1 tablespoon of olive oil and season with paprika, garlic powder, salt, and pepper.

3. In a separate bowl, toss cherry tomatoes, bell pepper slices, zucchini slices, and red onion slices with the remaining olive oil. Season with salt and pepper.

4. Spread the vegetables around the salmon fillets on the baking sheet.

5. Roast in the preheated oven for 15-20 minutes, or until the salmon is cooked through and flakes easily with a fork, and the vegetables are tender.

6. Remove from the oven and sprinkle with chopped fresh parsley, if desired.

7. Serve immediately with lemon wedges on the side.

Nutritional Information (per serving):

- Calories: 350

- Protein: 30g

- Sodium: 120mg

- Potassium: 900mg

- Total Fat: 20g

- Saturated Fat: 3g

- Cholesterol: 80mg

- Carbohydrates: 12g

- Fiber: 4g

- Sugars: 6g

Quinoa Stuffed Bell Peppers

Prep Time: 15 minutes

Cooking Time: 30 minutes

Serving Size: 1 stuffed pepper

Ingredients:

- 4 bell peppers (any color), halved and seeded

- 1 cup quinoa, rinsed

- 2 cups vegetable broth or water

- 1 tbsp olive oil

- 1 onion, diced

- 2 cloves garlic, minced

- 1 zucchini, diced

- 1 cup cherry tomatoes, halved

- 1 cup cooked black beans

- 1 tsp cumin

- 1 tsp chili powder

- Salt and pepper, to taste

- 1/2 cup shredded cheese (optional)

- Fresh cilantro, chopped, for garnish (optional)

Instructions:

1. Preheat oven to 375°F (190°C). Place the halved bell peppers in a baking dish, cut side up.

2. In a saucepan, combine quinoa and vegetable broth (or water) and bring to a boil. Reduce heat, cover, and simmer for 15 minutes, or until quinoa is cooked and liquid is absorbed.

3. In a separate skillet, heat olive oil over medium heat. Add diced onion and cook until translucent, about 5 minutes. Add minced garlic and cook for an additional 1-2 minutes.

4. Add diced zucchini to the skillet and cook for 3-4 minutes, until slightly softened.

5. Stir in cherry tomatoes, cooked black beans, cumin, chili powder, salt, and pepper. Cook for another 2-3 minutes.

6. Remove skillet from heat and stir in cooked quinoa until well combined.

7. Spoon the quinoa mixture into the halved bell peppers, dividing it evenly among them.

8. If using, sprinkle shredded cheese over the stuffed peppers.

9. Cover the baking dish with aluminum foil and bake in the preheated oven for 20-25 minutes, or until the peppers are tender.

10. Remove from the oven and garnish with chopped fresh cilantro, if desired.

Nutritional Information (per serving):

- Calories: 280
- Protein: 10g
- Sodium: 400mg
- Potassium: 600mg
- Total Fat: 8g
- Saturated Fat: 2g
- Cholesterol: 5mg
- Carbohydrates: 40g
- Fiber: 8g
- Sugars: 6g

Turkey and Vegetable Stir-Fry

Prep Time: 15 minutes

Cooking Time: 15 minutes

Serving Size: 1 cup

Ingredients:

- 1 lb turkey breast, thinly sliced

- 2 tbsp soy sauce (or tamari for gluten-free)

- 1 tbsp rice vinegar

- 1 tbsp honey

- 1 tbsp sesame oil

- 2 cloves garlic, minced

- 1-inch piece of ginger, minced

- 1 onion, sliced

- 1 bell pepper, sliced

- 1 cup broccoli florets

- 1 cup snow peas

- 1 carrot, julienned

- Cooked brown rice or quinoa, for serving

- Sesame seeds, for garnish (optional)

- Sliced green onions, for garnish (optional)

Instructions:

1. In a small bowl, whisk together soy sauce, rice vinegar, honey, and sesame oil to make the stir-fry sauce. Set aside.

2. Heat a large skillet or wok over medium-high heat. Add the turkey slices and cook until browned and cooked through about 5-6 minutes. Remove from skillet and set aside.

3. In the same skillet, add minced garlic and ginger, and sauté for 1 minute until fragrant.

4. Add sliced onion, bell pepper, broccoli florets, snow peas, and julienned carrot to the skillet. Stir-fry for 3-4 minutes until vegetables are tender-crisp.

5. Return the cooked turkey to the skillet and pour the stir-fry sauce over the turkey and vegetables. Stir well to coat everything evenly in the sauce.

6. Cook for an additional 2-3 minutes, stirring occasionally, until the sauce has thickened slightly.

7. Remove from heat and serve the turkey and vegetable stir-fry over cooked brown rice or quinoa.

8. Garnish with sesame seeds and sliced green onions, if desired.

Nutritional Information (per serving):

- Calories: 250

- Protein: 30g

- Sodium: 600mg

- Potassium: 700mg

- Total Fat: 5g

- Saturated Fat: 1g

- Cholesterol: 60mg

- Carbohydrates: 20g

- Fiber: 5g

- Sugars: 8g

Vegetarian Lentil Shepherd's Pie

Prep Time: 20 minutes

Cooking Time: 30 minutes

Serving Size: 1 slice

Ingredients:

- 2 cups green lentils, cooked

- 2 tbsp olive oil

- 1 onion, diced

- 2 cloves garlic, minced

- 2 carrots, diced

- 2 celery stalks, diced

- 1 cup frozen peas

- 1 cup frozen corn

- 2 tbsp tomato paste

- 1 tbsp Worcestershire sauce (optional)

- 1 tsp dried thyme

- 1 tsp dried rosemary

- Salt and pepper, to taste

- 4 cups mashed sweet potatoes

- Fresh parsley, chopped, for garnish (optional)

Instructions:

1. Preheat oven to 375°F (190°C). Grease a 9x13-inch baking dish with olive oil.

2. In a large skillet, heat olive oil over medium heat. Add diced onion and cook until translucent, about 5 minutes. Add minced garlic and cook for an additional 1-2 minutes.

3. Add diced carrots and celery to the skillet and cook for 5-7 minutes, until softened.

4. Stir in cooked green lentils, frozen peas, frozen corn, tomato paste, Worcestershire sauce (if using), dried thyme, dried rosemary, salt, and pepper. Cook for another 2-3 minutes until heated through.

5. Transfer the lentil mixture to the prepared baking dish and spread it out evenly.

6. Top the lentil mixture with mashed sweet potatoes, spreading them out evenly to cover the lentil mixture completely.

7. Bake in the preheated oven for 25-30 minutes, or until the sweet potato topping is lightly golden and the filling is bubbling around the edges.

8. Remove from the oven and let cool for a few minutes before slicing.

9. Garnish with chopped fresh parsley, if desired, before serving.

Nutritional Information (per serving):

- Calories: 320

- Protein: 12g

- Sodium: 400mg

- Potassium: 900mg

- Total Fat: 6g

- Saturated Fat: 1g

- Cholesterol: 0mg

- Carbohydrates: 55g

- Fiber: 12g

- Sugars: 12g

Salmon and Asparagus Foil Packets

Prep Time: 10 minutes

Cooking Time: 20 minutes

Serving Size: 1 packet

Ingredients:

- 4 salmon fillets

- 1 bunch asparagus, trimmed

- 2 cloves garlic, minced

- 2 tbsp olive oil

- 1 lemon, thinly sliced

- Fresh dill, chopped, for garnish

- Salt and pepper, to taste

Instructions:

1. Preheat oven to 375°F (190°C). Cut four large pieces of aluminum foil, about 12x18 inches each.

2. Place a salmon fillet in the center of each piece of foil. Season with minced garlic, salt, and pepper.

3. Arrange trimmed asparagus spears around each salmon fillet. Drizzle olive oil over the salmon and asparagus.

4. Place a few slices of lemon on top of each salmon fillet.

5. Fold the edges of the foil over the salmon and asparagus to create a packet, sealing tightly.

6. Place the foil packets on a baking sheet and bake in the preheated oven for 15-20 minutes, or until the salmon is cooked through and the asparagus is tender.

7. Carefully open the foil packets and transfer the salmon and asparagus to serving plates.

8. Garnish with chopped fresh dill before serving.

Nutritional Information (per serving):

- Calories: 280

- Protein: 30g

- Sodium: 100mg

- Potassium: 800mg

- Total Fat: 15g

- Saturated Fat: 2g

- Cholesterol: 80mg

- Carbohydrates: 5g

- Fiber: 2g

- Sugars: 2g

30-Day Meal Plan

Here's a 30-day meal plan using the provided recipes:

Day 1:

- Breakfast: Blueberry Almond Overnight Oats

- Lunch: Grilled Chicken Salad with Balsamic Vinaigrette

- Dinner: Grilled Lemon Herb Chicken

Day 2:

- Breakfast: Spinach and Feta Egg Muffins

- Lunch: Turkey and Avocado Wrap

- Dinner: Baked Salmon with Asparagus

Day 3:

- Breakfast: Quinoa Breakfast Bowl

- Lunch: Salmon and Quinoa Bowl

- Dinner: Stuffed Bell Peppers with Quinoa and Black Beans

Day 4:

- Breakfast: Avocado Toast with Poached Egg

- Lunch: Quinoa and Black Bean Salad

- Dinner: Grilled Lemon Garlic Shrimp Skewers

Day 5:

- Breakfast: Greek Yogurt Parfait

- Lunch: Grilled Vegetable Quesadilla

- Dinner: Turkey and Vegetable Stir-Fry

Day 6:

- Breakfast: Sweet Potato Breakfast Hash

- Lunch: Egg and Veggie Stir-Fry

- Dinner: Salmon with Roasted Vegetables

Day 7:

- Breakfast: Whole Grain Pancakes

- Lunch: Salmon Avocado Salad

- Dinner: Quinoa Stuffed Bell Peppers

Day 8:

- Breakfast: Spinach and Mushroom Omelette

- Lunch: Turkey and Vegetable Wrap

- Dinner: Vegetarian Lentil Shepherd's Pie

Day 9:

- Breakfast: Avocado Toast with Poached Egg

- Lunch: Greek Chicken Salad

- Dinner: Salmon and Asparagus Foil Packets

Day 10:

- Breakfast: Quinoa Breakfast Bowl

- Lunch: Quinoa Salad with Chickpeas and Avocado

- Dinner: Grilled Lemon Herb Chicken

Day 11:

- Breakfast: Blueberry Almond Overnight Oats

- Lunch: Grilled Vegetable Quesadilla

- Dinner: Baked Salmon with Asparagus

Day 12:

- Breakfast: Spinach and Feta Egg Muffins

- Lunch: Turkey and Vegetable Wrap

- Dinner: Stuffed Bell Peppers with Quinoa and Black Beans

Day 13:

- Breakfast: Greek Yogurt Parfait

- Lunch: Egg and Veggie Stir-Fry

- Dinner: Grilled Lemon Garlic Shrimp Skewers

Day 14:

- Breakfast: Sweet Potato Breakfast Hash

- Lunch: Salmon Avocado Salad

- Dinner: Turkey and Vegetable Stir-Fry

Day 15:

- Breakfast: Whole Grain Pancakes

- Lunch: Quinoa and Black Bean Salad

- Dinner: Quinoa Stuffed Bell Peppers

Day 16:

- Breakfast: Spinach and Mushroom Omelette

- Lunch: Greek Chicken Salad

- Dinner: Salmon and Asparagus Foil Packets

Day 17:

- Breakfast: Avocado Toast with Poached Egg

- Lunch: Grilled Vegetable Quesadilla

- Dinner: Grilled Lemon Herb Chicken

Day 18:

- Breakfast: Quinoa Breakfast Bowl

- Lunch: Turkey and Avocado Wrap

- Dinner: Stuffed Bell Peppers with Quinoa and Black Beans

Day 19:

- Breakfast: Blueberry Almond Overnight Oats

- Lunch: Quinoa Salad with Chickpeas and Avocado

- Dinner: Baked Salmon with Asparagus

Day 20:

- Breakfast: Spinach and Feta Egg Muffins

- Lunch: Salmon and Quinoa Bowl

- Dinner: Turkey and Vegetable Stir-Fry

Day 21:

- Breakfast: Greek Yogurt Parfait

- Lunch: Egg and Veggie Stir-Fry

- Dinner: Grilled Lemon Garlic Shrimp Skewers

Day 22:

- Breakfast: Sweet Potato Breakfast Hash

- Lunch: Turkey and Vegetable Wrap

- Dinner: Salmon with Roasted Vegetables

Day 23:

- Breakfast: Whole Grain Pancakes

- Lunch: Salmon Avocado Salad

- Dinner: Quinoa Stuffed Bell Peppers

Day 24:

- Breakfast: Avocado Toast with Poached Egg

- Lunch: Grilled Vegetable Quesadilla

- Dinner: Vegetarian Lentil Shepherd's Pie

Day 25:

- Breakfast: Quinoa Breakfast Bowl

- Lunch: Greek Chicken Salad

- Dinner: Salmon and Asparagus Foil Packets

Day 26:

- Breakfast: Blueberry Almond Overnight Oats

- Lunch: Grilled Chicken Salad with Balsamic Vinaigrette

- Dinner: Grilled Lemon Herb Chicken

Day 27:

- Breakfast: Spinach and Feta Egg Muffins

- Lunch: Turkey and Avocado Wrap

- Dinner: Baked Salmon with Asparagus

Day 28:

- Breakfast: Quinoa Breakfast Bowl

- Lunch: Salmon and Quinoa Bowl

- Dinner: Stuffed Bell Peppers with Quinoa and Black Beans

Day 29:

- Breakfast: Avocado Toast with Poached Egg

- Lunch: Quinoa and Black Bean Salad

- Dinner: Grilled Lemon Garlic Shrimp Skewers

Day 30:

- Breakfast: Greek Yogurt Parfait

- Lunch: Egg and Veggie Stir-Fry

- Dinner: Turkey and Vegetable Stir-Fry

CHAPTER 7

ADAPTING THE DIET TO YOUR LIFESTYLE

Eating Out and Social Events

Maintaining your dietary goals while eating out or attending social events can be challenging when following the Metabolic Confusion Diet. However, with careful planning and mindful choices, you can navigate these situations without compromising your progress.

One effective strategy is to research menu options before dining out. Many restaurants now provide nutritional information online, allowing you to make informed choices in advance. Look for dishes that align with the principles of the Metabolic Confusion Diet, such as those featuring lean protein sources, whole grains, and plenty of vegetables. Additionally, don't hesitate to request substitutions or modifications to accommodate your dietary preferences.

Another approach is to practice portion control when dining out. Restaurant servings are often oversized, which can lead to excessive calorie intake. Consider sharing entrees with a dining partner or opting for a half portion to avoid overeating. Pay attention to your hunger and fullness cues, and stop eating when you feel satisfied rather than finishing everything on your plate.

During social events, such as parties or gatherings, you may encounter tempting foods and drinks. While occasional indulgence is acceptable, it's essential to maintain moderation. Fill your plate with nutrient-dense options like fruits, vegetables, and lean proteins, and limit your consumption of high-calorie, low-nutrient foods.

Effective communication is key when navigating social situations. Inform your friends, family, or hosts about your dietary preferences and goals so they can accommodate your needs. Don't hesitate to ask questions about ingredients or preparation methods if you're uncertain. Most people will be understanding and supportive of your choices.

Remember to strike a balance between adhering to your dietary goals and enjoying social occasions. By making mindful choices and planning, you can successfully manage eating out and social events while following the Metabolic Confusion Diet.

Combining Metabolic Confusion with Intermittent Fasting

Intermittent fasting, a dietary approach involving alternating periods of eating and fasting, has gained popularity in recent years. When combined with the Metabolic Confusion Diet, intermittent fasting can enhance metabolic flexibility, promote fat loss, and improve overall health outcomes.

One common method of intermittent fasting is the 16/8 protocol, which entails fasting for 16 hours and eating during an 8-hour window each day. This approach can be seamlessly integrated into the Metabolic Confusion Diet by adjusting your eating schedule. For example, you might skip breakfast and commence your eating window later in the day, allowing for larger meals in the afternoon and evening.

Another option is the 5:2 method, where you eat normally for five days of the week and restrict calorie intake to 500-600 calories on two non-consecutive days. On fasting days, focus on consuming nutrient-dense, low-calorie foods like vegetables, lean proteins, and broth-based soups to stay satiated and minimize hunger.

You can also vary your fasting and eating patterns throughout the week to incorporate metabolic confusion principles. Alternate between different fasting protocols on different days, such as fasting for 16 hours one day and 18 hours the next. Occasionally, include longer fasts lasting 24 hours or more.

It's crucial to listen to your body and adjust your fasting schedule based on your individual needs and preferences. Some individuals may find intermittent fasting challenging initially, so start gradually and increase fasting durations over time.

Physical Activity Recommendations

Regular physical activity is vital for optimizing metabolic health, supporting weight management, and enhancing overall well-being in conjunction with the Metabolic Confusion Diet. Here are some recommendations for incorporating exercise into your lifestyle:

- Engage in a variety of cardiovascular exercises, strength training, and flexibility exercises to promote overall fitness. Activities like walking, jogging, cycling, or swimming improve heart health and burn calories, while strength training exercises build muscle mass and metabolism. Flexibility exercises such as yoga enhance mobility and reduce injury risk.

- Choose activities that you enjoy and that align with your lifestyle. Whether it's dancing, hiking, playing sports, or attending group fitness classes, select activities that you find enjoyable and are likely to sustain long-term.

- Set realistic and achievable fitness goals. Whether it's walking for 30 minutes a day, strength training three times a week, or working towards a specific fitness milestone, clear goals help maintain motivation and focus. Begin with manageable goals and gradually increase intensity and duration as your fitness improves.

- Integrate movement into your daily routine whenever possible. Opt for stairs over elevators, walk or bike instead of driving short distances, and break up prolonged sitting with brief activity breaks throughout the day.

- Prioritize rest and recovery to prevent overtraining and injury. Incorporate one or two rest days per week, and include activities like stretching or yoga to relax muscles and enhance recovery.

- Stay hydrated and consume a balanced diet rich in lean proteins, whole grains, fruits, and vegetables to support physical activity goals.

By incorporating regular physical activity into your routine, you can maximize the benefits of the Metabolic Confusion Diet and achieve your health and fitness objectives effectively.

Monitoring Your Progress

Tracking your progress is a crucial aspect of any dietary or lifestyle change, including the Metabolic Confusion Diet. By monitoring your food intake, physical activity, and relevant metrics, you can evaluate progress, identify areas for improvement, and make necessary adjustments to achieve your goals.

One effective method is maintaining a food diary or utilizing a mobile app to record meals, snacks, and beverages throughout the day. Tracking your food intake promotes awareness of eating habits, helps identify patterns or triggers leading to unhealthy choices, and enables adjustments accordingly.

In addition to food tracking, monitor factors such as energy levels, mood, sleep quality, and physical symptoms. Observe how you feel before and after meals, sleep patterns, and overall health changes.

Keep a log of your physical activity and exercise routines, including type, duration, intensity, and notable achievements. Monitoring physical activity ensures accountability to fitness goals and confirms adequate movement for health and fitness objectives.

CHAPTER 8

OVERCOMING CHALLENGES AND STAYING MOTIVATED

Common Pitfalls and How to Avoid Them

Embarking on any diet plan, such as the Metabolic Confusion Diet, presents challenges. Recognizing these pitfalls and learning how to overcome them is crucial for long-term success. Here are some common pitfalls and strategies to avoid them:

Lack of Preparation: One of the biggest challenges is being unprepared for your dietary journey. Without planning, it's easy to make unhealthy food choices when hunger strikes or when faced with limited options.

- *Solution*: Set aside time each week to plan and prepare meals. Create a weekly meal plan, make a shopping list, and batch-cook healthy recipes in advance. Having nutritious meals and snacks readily available makes it easier to stick to your dietary goals, especially when life gets busy.

Social Pressure: Social gatherings and peer influence can derail even the most committed individuals. The temptation to indulge in unhealthy foods or drinks can be hard to resist in social settings.

- *Solution*: Communicate your dietary goals and preferences with friends, family, and colleagues. Let them know why you're following the Metabolic Confusion Diet and how they can support you. Bringing your healthy dish to gatherings or offering to host can give you more control over the menu. Remember, moderation is key when indulging occasionally.

Emotional Eating: Turning to food for comfort or stress relief can lead to mindless eating and unhealthy habits. Emotional triggers like boredom, anxiety, or sadness can hinder your progress.

- *Solution*: Find alternative coping mechanisms for dealing with emotions, such as journaling, meditation, exercise, or talking to a friend. Practice mindfulness when eating by paying attention to hunger and fullness cues and choosing nourishing foods that satisfy both your body and mind.

All-or-Nothing Mentality: Striving for perfection and expecting instant results can lead to disappointment and frustration. Progress takes time, and setbacks are part of the journey.

- *Solution*: Shift your mindset to one of flexibility and self-compassion. Focus on making small, sustainable changes rather than aiming for perfection. Celebrate progress, no matter how small, and learn from setbacks without dwelling on them.

Unrealistic Expectations: Unrealistic expectations about weight loss or body image can lead to disappointment and feelings of failure.

- *Solution*: Set realistic, achievable goals focused on health and well-being rather than just the number on the scale. Celebrate non-scale victories like increased energy or improved mood. Remember, everyone's journey is unique, and progress looks different for everyone.

Dealing with Plateaus

Experiencing a plateau, where weight loss or progress stalls, is common on any diet plan, including the Metabolic Confusion Diet. Plateaus can be frustrating, but they're also an opportunity to reassess your approach and make necessary adjustments. Here are some strategies for breaking through plateaus:

Review Your Eating Habits: Take a closer look at your dietary habits. Are you still following the principles of the Metabolic Confusion Diet? Are you eating balanced meals with lean proteins, whole grains, and plenty of fruits and vegetables?

- *Solution*: Keep a food diary to track your meals and assess whether you're consuming more calories than you realize. Look for areas where you can make improvements, such as reducing portion sizes or cutting back on added sugars.

Reevaluate Your Exercise Routine: It may be time to shake up your exercise routine if you've hit a plateau. Your body can adapt to repetitive workouts, leading to diminished results over time.

- *Solution*: Incorporate variety into your exercise regimen by trying new activities or changing the intensity or duration of your workouts. Strength training can help build muscle mass and boost metabolism.

Manage Stress Levels: Chronic stress can interfere with weight loss by increasing cortisol levels and promoting fat storage.

- *Solution*: Incorporate stress-reducing activities into your daily routine, such as meditation or yoga. Prioritize self-care to promote relaxation and well-being.

Ensure Adequate Sleep: Lack of sleep can disrupt hormonal balance and metabolism, making it harder to lose weight.

- *Solution*: Aim for 7-9 hours of quality sleep per night. Establish a consistent sleep schedule and create a relaxing bedtime routine.

Stay Patient and Persistent: Plateaus are a normal part of the weight loss journey. Stay committed to your goals and trust the process.

- *Solution*: Focus on making sustainable lifestyle changes rather than chasing quick fixes. Celebrate progress, no matter how small, and stay patient as you work toward your goals.

Keeping Motivated Over Time

Maintaining motivation is crucial for long-term success in the Metabolic Confusion Diet. Here are some strategies for staying motivated:

Set Clear Goals: Establish specific, measurable goals that align with your values and priorities.

- *Solution*: Write down your goals and track your progress regularly. Celebrate achievements along the way to stay motivated.

Find Your Why: Identify your reasons for following the Metabolic Confusion Diet and prioritize your health and well-being.

- *Solution*: Reflect on the benefits of achieving your goals and keep your reasons front and center as a reminder of why you started your journey.

Create a Support System: Surround yourself with supportive friends and family who can cheer you on.

- *Solution*: Share your goals and progress with others and seek out like-minded individuals for support and encouragement.

Practice Self-Compassion: Be kind to yourself and avoid self-criticism.

- *Solution*: Practice self-care activities that nourish your body and mind. Take breaks when needed and ask for help when feeling overwhelmed.

Stay Flexible and Adaptive: Be willing to adapt your approach based on feedback from your body and progress.

- *Solution*: Experiment with different strategies and adjust your plan as needed to support your goals.

CHAPTER 9

CONCLUSION

In conclusion, embarking on the Metabolic Confusion Diet journey requires dedication, perseverance, and a willingness to adapt. Throughout this book, we've explored the principles of the Metabolic Confusion Diet, including its emphasis on varying macronutrient intake, incorporating nutrient-dense foods, and implementing strategic fasting periods. We've delved into the science behind metabolic flexibility and how it can promote fat loss, improve metabolic health, and enhance overall well-being.

As we've discussed, the Metabolic Confusion Diet offers a flexible and sustainable approach to weight loss and metabolic health. By cycling between periods of higher and lower calorie intake and varying macronutrient ratios, the body is forced to adapt, leading to increased metabolic flexibility and improved fat-burning efficiency. Additionally, strategic fasting periods can further enhance metabolic function, promote autophagy, and support overall health.

Throughout the book, we've addressed common challenges and pitfalls that individuals may encounter on their Metabolic Confusion Diet journey. From overcoming social pressure and emotional eating to breaking through plateaus and staying motivated over time, we've provided practical strategies and solutions to help readers navigate these obstacles and stay on track with their goals.

One of the key themes that emerged is the importance of preparation and planning. By setting aside time each week to plan and prepare meals, individuals can ensure they have nutritious options readily available, making it easier to stick to their dietary goals even in the face of busy schedules or social events. Additionally, establishing a support system and practicing self-compassion is essential for maintaining motivation and resilience in the face of setbacks or challenges.

As individuals progress on their Metabolic Confusion Diet journey, it's important to remember that progress may not always be linear. Plateaus are a natural part of the process, and setbacks are to be expected. By staying patient, persistent, and adaptable, individuals can navigate these challenges and continue moving forward toward their health and wellness goals.

In addition to dietary changes, we've emphasized the importance of incorporating regular physical activity into one's routine. Exercise not only supports weight loss and metabolic health but also enhances mood, energy levels, and overall well-being. Finding activities that are enjoyable and sustainable is key to long-term adherence and success.

Finally, monitoring progress and celebrating achievements along the way is crucial for maintaining motivation and momentum. Whether it's tracking food intake, measuring physical activity, or assessing changes in energy levels and mood, regular self-assessment can provide valuable insights and feedback to guide one's journey.

In essence, the Metabolic Confusion Diet is not just a temporary fix or quick solution but rather a lifestyle approach to health and wellness. By embracing flexibility, balance, and self-compassion, individuals can cultivate a positive relationship with food, enhance metabolic function, and achieve sustainable weight loss and overall well-being. As individuals continue on their journey, it's important to stay curious, open-minded, and willing to experiment with different strategies to find what works best for their unique needs and preferences.